What People Are Saying About *The Gold Coast Cure* . . .

"In this eminently sensible and useful book, Dr. Andrew Larson and exercise specialist Ivy Larson offer sound guidance for lasting health benefits."

David L. Katz, M.D., MPH, FACPM, FACP, author, *The Way to Eat,*
associate clinical professor and director of Medical Studies in Public Health at Yale

"Finally, a diet book that I would recommend to friends, family and clients. Dr. Larson and his wife, Ivy, are careful to separate scientific fact from scientific opinion. They hit the mark with their philosophy of nutrition first, medication second—addressing the body as whole, not individual parts. The Larsons' advice is practical, encouraging a wide variety of whole, naturally nutrient-dense foods and avoiding excess intake while still allowing for the occasional sweet treat to please the palate."

Lona Sandon, M.Ed., R.D., assistant professor, clinical nutrition, UT Southwestern
Medical Center; spokesperson, the American Dietetic Association

"*The Gold Coast Cure* is about transformation. . . . This book will indeed transform the paradigm of illness and health for many, opening new doors to allow health to flourish."

David Perlmutter, M.D., FACN, author, *The Better Brain Book*

"The American obsession with fad diets is leading to many health problems. *The Gold Coast Cure's* anti-inflammatory diet is based on delicious, healing foods instead of the gimmicks that create inflammation and disease. In a nation where obesity and disease are rampant, it's critical to read this book to understand how certain foods cause many of the weight problems and diseases that plague you and those you love."

Marci Page Sloane, M.S., R.D., LD/N, CDE,
author, *The Diet Game*

"Coming from a lifetime of fitness teaching and education, it's great to find a book that brings together an effective and sound nutritional and exercise plan. *The Gold Coast Cure* will help people master the lifestyle changes needed to improve and maintain optimal wellness, as well as reverse many of the chronic diseases that have become common today."

Joy Prouty, certified fitness professional, American College of
Sports Medicine, American Council for Exercise,
Aerobic Fitness Association of America
and Reebok University Master Trainer

"Over the years, I have paid great attention to my health—not only for my quality of golf but for my quality of life. I have worked with some of the world's finest from the fields of fitness and nutrition. A common link among people considered the best in their chosen fields is they give you guidance today but, more important, hope for tomorrow. This is Andy and Ivy's goal with *The Gold Coast Cure*. I applaud them for reaching out to everyone in need of a lifestyle change, but mainly to those battling chronic diseases who are searching for help and hope."

Jack Nicklaus, golf legend

"In *The Gold Coast Cure*, the Larsons will teach you a science-based program that promotes lifelong health. Whether you are fighting a disease or working on staying healthy, this program will make you feel better."

Susan M. Kleiner, Ph.D, R.D., FACN, CNS, author, *Power Eating*

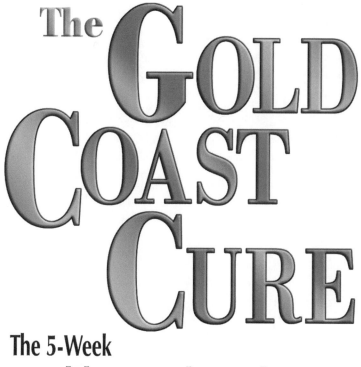

The GOLD COAST CURE

The 5-Week
Health & Body Makeover

Andrew Larson, M.D.
Ivy Ingram Larson

Health Communications, Inc.
Deerfield Beach, Florida

www.hcibooks.com

Library of Congress Cataloging-in-Publication Data
is available from the Library of Congress

©2005 Andrew Larson, M.D., and Ivy Ingram Larson
ISBN 0-7573-0235-1

Publisher: Health Communications, Inc.
3201 S.W. 15th Street
Deerfield Beach, FL 33442–8190

Cover design by Larissa Hise Henoch
Inside book design by Lawna Patterson Oldfield

In loving memory of our dear friend
Alexander John (A. J.) Cotsalas.
We miss you and will always remember you.

Contents

PART ONE: Positive Changes Mean Positive Results: Using the Cure to Heal Yourself

PART TWO: Eating for Weight Loss and Health: The Foods That Slim and Heal

PART THREE: The Gold Coast Diet and Lifestyle Plan

PART FOUR: The Gold Coast Cookbook

Acknowledgments

So many people helped bring this book together. We are sincerely grateful to them all for their commitment, time and support.

We can't thank Ivy's mom, Gail Ingram, enough for her enthusiasm from day one. It was really Gail who encouraged us to follow through with our plan to write this book. We want to thank her also for her never-ending willingness to pitch in and help *whenever* needed. Gail was always eager to lend a hand, from helping develop, test . . . and re-test . . . various recipes, to trying out exercise routines, to saving the day at the last minute, and so much more! Thank you so much, Mom, for the time and dedication you have put into this project.

We also want to extend an *enormous* thank-you to Ivy's father, Norman Ingram, for his tremendous generosity throughout Andy's residency. We could not have completed this project without your financial help. You will never know how much we both appreciate it, Dad!

We owe a very big thank-you to Andy's parents, Ken and Elaine Larson, who have both been so incredibly helpful throughout the many difficult years of residency and through the years it has taken us to complete this project. We can't express how much we appreciate the countless times and ways you have come to our rescue. Many, many thanks to you both!

At Health Communications, we owe executive editor Allison Janse a page of her own! Allison, you believed in our book from the very beginning: We thank you so much for your dedication to our project and for your invaluable insight. You succeeded in translating our work into something everyone can understand and use. Your thoroughness, commitment and backing have been invaluable! To the director of communications, Kim Weiss, because of your enthusiasm, hard work and support you not only found the doors, you opened them too! We can't thank you enough for going the extra miles on this project! To our publisher, Peter Vegso, we will always be indebted to you for giving us the opportunity to make our dream come true. Your faith in us is sincerely appreciated. We will be forever grateful! And a heartfelt thank you to all of the many other people at Health Communications who worked so hard to pull this book together.

A very special thank-you to our dear friend Erin Glynn for giving us the opportunity to hold our first "5 Week Shape-Up" and for encouraging us so wholeheartedly through the early years. A sincere thank-you to our friend Regina Gausepohl who was a driving force behind getting our program into the medical community. And of course, a very big thank-you to all of the participants in our first "5 Week Shape-Up" class at the Atlantic Club in Red Bank, New Jersey. Thank you all for believing in us and in our program.

Thank you to Dr. William Sheremata for setting Ivy in the right direction from the beginning. To one of Ivy's best friends, Carla Canedo, thank you so much for sticking your neck out for us in the early stages. Jack Nicklaus, thank you for trusting us and helping us when we needed it most.

And last, but not least, we want to thank our dear son Blake for his significant contribution in making the Cure a family plan. We love you so much!

Foreword

Sixteenth-century physician Paracelsus stated, "Medicine is not only a science; it is also an art. It does not consist of compounding pills and plasters; it deals with the very processes of life, which must be understood before they may be guided." In today's world, many of us—patients and physicians alike—feel the art of medicine has been lost.

For many reasons, the physician's involvement in understanding vitally important health issues often takes a back seat to a reflexive response that culminates in writing a prescription after a ten-minute office visit. While the usefulness of pharmaceutical drugs in a variety of medical conditions cannot be disputed, overreliance on this specific modality is just one of the shortcomings of modern Western medicine.

Another problem confronting physicians and patients alike is the segregation of health-care practitioners based upon their approaches to health and disease. Nowadays, physicians who incorporate nutritional counseling and lifestyle modifications, like recommending adequate sleep and exercise, are labeled as practicing "alternative" or "holistic" medicine, terms typically used to differentiate these approaches from traditional medicine. Webster's dictionary defines the word "traditional" as ". . . communicated from ancestors to descendants . . . transmitted from age to age." Indeed, important cornerstones of health that have been part of the human experience for millennia are often overlooked in modern medical practice.

Andy and Ivy Larson, the authors of *The Gold Coast Cure,* experienced this firsthand when Ivy began experiencing debilitating symptoms of fatigue, numbness and muscle weakness at the age of twenty-two. One physician told her that her symptoms were due to anxiety; another told her that these symptoms were normal. She persisted, though, and found a doctor who provided the right diagnosis: multiple sclerosis. Fortunately, this physician practiced the "art" of medicine. He didn't just write her a prescription. He took the time to listen to Ivy; he recognized her background in fitness and knew she was highly motivated to change her health for the better. He suggested she modify her diet instead of taking drugs, an idea that seemed radical to some, including her husband, Andy, who was completing medical school at the time.

The Gold Coast Cure is about transformation, first the transformation of a physician and his ailing wife, and second the transformation of the reader. This book will indeed transform the paradigm of illness and health for many, opening new doors to allow health to flourish while illness fades.

While *The Gold Coast Cure* is founded on trusted principles that have been part of the human experience for ages, Andy and Ivy support these timeless principles with the most state-of-the-art scientific research. Truly then, this well-grounded approach to health and well-being promises readers not another dangerous fad or quick-fix approach: It offers readers a powerful and proactive plan for a lifetime of health and wellness.

David Perlmutter, M.D., FACN
board-certified neurologist;
fellow, American College of Nutrition
author, *The Better Brain Book*

Introduction

Ivy's Story: How I Defeated
Multiple Sclerosis by Changing My Diet

If you saw me chasing after my four-year-old son in the park or running with my husband on the beach you'd probably think I've always been healthy. You'd never guess that as recently as seven years ago, I struggled to walk up a flight of stairs due to weakness in my right leg, I was often incontinent, and I could barely make it through the day because I was constantly exhausted. At the age of twenty-two I felt like I was eighty-two, and I was seriously worried that I would never feel better.

Ironically, at the time I became ill, I was working as a health and fitness instructor at a medical center on the Gold Coast of Florida. I loved my job, which included evaluating patients, developing exercise prescriptions to help them regain mobility and teaching fitness classes. Many of my clients had serious health conditions like arthritis, heart disease, osteoporosis, diabetes and obesity, and I felt truly rewarded by my role in helping them back to health.

Although I worked out regularly, I didn't pay much attention to what I put in my mouth. I was blessed with a fast metabolism, and I happily took advantage of it: My all-time favorite food was ice cream. I pretty much ate what I wanted, then hit the gym. I looked fit and healthy, but that was far from the truth.

I suddenly began suffering from bladder infections—as many as three a month. I constantly felt the urge to run to the bathroom, and I literally planned my days around access to a toilet.

I spent an entire summer visiting physician after physician, yet couldn't obtain an accurate diagnosis. One doctor told me I was a "nervous-natured" girl, another told me to sit in a hot bath four to six times a day to relax, and another insisted that using the bathroom twenty times a day was normal!

Things got progressively worse. My right leg became numb, and I lost considerable strength in my right hip muscle, making it difficult for me to lift my leg. Teaching exercise class was nearly impossible, and I was becoming more depressed with each passing day.

One night, thinking that another bladder infection was beginning, I followed doctor's instructions and drank nearly four cups of cranberry juice and water. Thirty minutes into *The Horse Whisperer*, I thought my bladder was going to explode. I ran to the ladies' room, but couldn't go. I wound up in the emergency room, and I left the hospital wearing a catheter. While I knew something was terribly wrong, I was terrified to imagine what it was.

Still wearing the catheter, I traveled with my parents to the University of Miami to obtain a diagnosis. After extensive testing by a prominent urologist, I was referred to Dr. William Sheremata, a world-class neurologist. Frustrated at what seemed like another dead-end, I wondered how a brain doctor was going to fix my bladder.

After sending me for MRI scans of my head and spinal cord, Dr. Sheremata did have the answer, but it wasn't what I wanted to hear: "Multiple sclerosis," he said without hesitation. I sat in his pea-green office in a daze, listening to him enumerate the symptoms of the diagnosis, many of which I already had: bladder problems, visual disturbances, depression, impaired memory, loss of mental clarity, debilitating fatigue, weakness, paralysis, inability to swallow, numbness and tingling in the extremities, difficulty walking, loss of coordination, and overwhelming dizziness.

I thought my life was over. The disease sounded like a living nightmare to me. Grim thoughts flooded my mind: *Would I ever be able to have children? Would I always need to wear a catheter? Was I going to end up in a wheelchair?*

As frustrated and frightened as I was about my symptoms, I learned that many multiple sclerosis (MS) patients suffer from problems far worse than mine. An increasingly common disease of the central nervous system, MS tends to strike at an early age, and although the course of MS is highly unpredictable, the disease can ultimately result in significant disability.[1]

After the initial shock wore off, my doctor gave me hope by telling me that MS can be controlled by adhering to a healthful lifestyle. He gave me the option of taking a disease-modifying drug to treat the

Dr. Swank's Diet

Dr. Roy L. Swank's research dates back to 1948, long before modern disease-modifying MS drugs were available. Over the course of a nearly fifty-year career, Dr. Swank worked directly with thousands of MS patients, and his diet has been proven to reduce the frequency and severity of exacerbations in MS patients. After a period of five years, study patients who followed his diet were actually better off functionally than when they were first diagnosed with multiple sclerosis. At twenty years, most of the control group patients were unable to walk, whereas the typical Swank diet patient was fully mobile and experiencing only mild symptoms.

The current edition of Dr. Swank's book, *The Multiple Sclerosis Diet Book* (1987, Doubleday), provides irrefutable evidence that diet does in fact improve the symptoms of multiple sclerosis. Large studies published in prestigious medical journals such as the *Journal of Neurology, Neurosurgery, and Psychiatry*,[2] smaller-scale studies published in less widely known journals,[3] basic science studies,[4] and high-quality epidemiologic studies[5] have all linked the improvement of real-life human (not rat, not mouse, not chimpanzee) multiple sclerosis with dietary changes.

MS, but he also advised me to try the Dr. Swank diet for multiple sclerosis. I decided to hold off on the medication and try the diet first.

At the time of my diagnosis, my future husband, Andy, was studying at one of the top three medical schools in the country. Despite his medical training, Andy questioned my decision to try nutritional therapy instead of prescription medication; he'd never heard about treating MS with diet, and he was skeptical. He spent hours at the University of Pennsylvania's medical library reading all of the available literature. Only then, to his astonishment, was he able to confirm that the Swank diet did in fact have merit.

Although it seems like common sense that anyone suffering from chronic illness should maintain a healthful lifestyle, many medical doctors remain highly suspicious of, or at least unimpressed with, nutritional therapies. Even though we view physicians as the ultimate authorities when it comes to health, the average medical student receives less than thirty hours of training in nutrition and no instruction in exercise therapy or nutritional supplementation. Most medical students graduate uninformed about these keys to good health unless they develop their own intellectual interest.

Although Andy and I were impressed with the results of the Swank program, I was having a difficult time sticking to the bland diet. Hoping that a more enjoyable program existed, we pored over countless medical and exercise science journals, reading everything we could about diet, exercise and MS. After extensive research, we discovered an irrefutable connection between the foods I was eating and my MS. Armed with this information, we developed an enjoyable eating plan consisting of healing, anti-inflammatory foods and a supplementation regimen that controlled my MS by fighting inflammation and keeping my immune system optimally fueled. I then customized an exercise program to rebuild my muscular strength and keep MS complications at bay. In the past I had worked with MS patients who were more disabled than they needed to be as a result of inactivity. Many of them had problems with balance, muscle atrophy, fatigue and weakness that could have been greatly improved with consistent resistance training exercise. Although I knew exercise alone wouldn't "cure" my MS, I knew a consistent program of strength training could dramatically improve my quality of life.

My health improved rapidly. First I noticed a dramatic increase in my strength and energy levels. The catheter was removed, and I have never experienced another bladder problem since that night I ended up in the emergency room. The awful sensations of urgency and frequency also diminished. I began waking up fewer times at night and holding my bladder for longer periods during the day. The incontinence stopped altogether, and the strength in my right hip returned.

As I noticed my health improving, I also noticed that I was falling in love with Andy. Luckily for me, he was feeling the same way. We were married several years later and when we vowed to love each other in sickness and health, we knew in our hearts we were speaking the truth.

Four years ago I gave birth to our incredibly healthy son, Blake, and never experienced a post-pregnancy flare-up that is so common among women with MS. It has been seven years now since I was diagnosed, and today I can honestly say I feel better than ever. Not only am I measurably stronger and healthier than I was at the time of my diagnosis, I no longer feel like my body is betraying me. I have stopped going to bed worrying if I will wake up in the morning with some horrible MS symptom. The physiological burden of MS is gone.

After witnessing firsthand how effective nutritional therapy was in fighting my inflammatory condition, Andy and I realized that our plan could treat other modern diseases because it combats two culprits that cause and exacerbate disease: inflammation and malnutrition. By reducing or eliminating these two problems, our Gold Coast

Cure could treat ten chronic diseases—arthritis, asthma, heart disease, allergies, fibromyalgia, type II diabetes, vascular dementia, obesity, osteoporosis and multiple sclerosis—as well as offer protection from certain types of cancer and improve cholesterol ratios.

After sharing our recommendations with friends and family, we brought our program to the public through a wellness class at the prestigious Atlantic Club in Red Bank, New Jersey. The class was advertised as a "5 Week Shape-Up" for club members who had health problems ranging from high cholesterol and high triglyceride levels to asthma, fibromyalgia, type II diabetes, obesity, MS and arthritis.

While we were confident we could help our clients, we weren't sure we could obtain measurable results for such a wide variety of conditions in just five weeks! As part of our first class, we performed extensive testing on every client, including a complete cholesterol profile, blood pressure testing, triglyceride testing, waist and hip measurements, and body fat analysis. For five weeks the class met three times a week for one hour.

The results were nothing less than astonishing: In as little as five weeks every client saw measurable improvements in not only their appearance but their health. Every single person lost weight, decreased their body fat percentage, and lost inches from either their waist or hips, or both. Every person who had high triglycerides saw a decrease; every person who suffered from an inflammation-mediated condition such as asthma, arthritis, multiple sclerosis or fibromyalgia enjoyed a marked improvement in their symptoms; and every person except for one saw improvements in their total cholesterol level and their overall cholesterol profile. For example:

• A fibromyalgia patient enjoyed significant improvement in her energy levels, sleep quality and relief from the pain and stiffness associated with her disease; her total cholesterol decreased from 208 to 179; she lost 2 inches from her waist and hips.

- A middle-aged woman decreased her cholesterol from 252 to 213 and lost 4 inches from her waist and hips.
- A fairly healthy fifty-five-year-old man joined the class hoping to reduce his high cholesterol level. Not only did his total cholesterol drop from 305 to 245, his "bad" LDL cholesterol dropped from 229 to 187 and he decreased his body fat from an already fit 17.2 percent to an even leaner 15 percent.
- A fifty-nine-year-old man lowered his body fat from 29.5 percent to 26 percent and lost 4 pounds. He lost 4½ inches from his waist and hips, lowered his cholesterol from 250 to 196, and lowered his triglycerides from 87 to 70.

One of our clients, a nurse who directs a prominent cardiac rehabilitation program, came to us hoping to improve severe arthritis symptoms. She'd been unable to cross her legs for years due to the

Nutritional Therapy First, Medication Second

Despite our emphasis on the lifestyle approach to disease management, we respect everything modern medicine has to offer. We're not opposed to medication for any of the chronic conditions our book targets. (If and when I need to take one of the disease-modifying drugs currently available to treat MS, I won't hesitate. However, my symptoms have been under excellent control since I began a program of nutritional therapy.) It's critical to recognize, however, that medicine alone will never give you optimal health. Medicine can only take you so far. By and large, medicines treat the *symptoms* of disease and not the *underlying problem*. Your body works as a whole, and you can't expect to treat one particular ailment with medicine and then sit back and enjoy optimal health. Medicines almost always have side effects, some of which are worse than the diseases they are designed to treat.

pain in her knees, she couldn't walk up a flight of stairs, and she could barely bend down to pick something up off the floor. Our initial blood work revealed her cholesterol level to be dangerously high. At the end of our five-week class, she was crossing her legs, climbing stairs easily and without pain, and walking miles a day on the streets of Manhattan! She lost seven pounds and decreased her body fat percentage from 33 percent to 28.5 percent. She was so impressed with these results she invited us to talk about the Gold Coast Cure with advanced practice nurses representing the Tri-State Society of the American Association of Cardiovascular and Pulmonary Rehabilitation. From there the word spread, and we've been presenting our program to patients and health care professionals ever since.

We wrote this book to share what we've learned with everyone who suffers from the chronic conditions we target. Having personally experienced the tragic consequences of lost hope, we want to share with you our message that things can improve. Our dear friend A. J., to whom this book is dedicated, also had MS. His physicians gave him medication, but they didn't give him a reason to think that he could feel better. They insisted that nutritional therapy was a waste of his time. Without a medical background, our friend had to rely on the MS "experts" for advice on how to control his disease. When his symptoms took a sharp turn for the worse, despite painful injections of a disease-modifying medication that was becoming increasingly ineffective, A. J. took his life at the age of thirty. We firmly believe A. J. would still be here today if he had been given the hope of a brighter future.

The Cure offers hope. Although we were initially devastated to learn about my MS, once we learned there was a blueprint for health that could slow or even reverse the progress of this debilitating disease, we became hopeful for our future. And there's hope for you, too. Whether you want to lose the last stubborn ten pounds, get your diabetes under control or simply have more energy to get through your days, the Cure can work for you.

Small Changes, Big Effects

You don't have to be ill to be on the Cure. This is a lifestyle plan that you can follow in sickness *and* in health because it prevents and reverses degenerative disease and whittles your waistline. By following the Cure you'll not only improve your health, you'll also improve your appearance.

Within five weeks, you and your physician alike will see real results. You will appreciate a definite difference in the way you feel and the way you look. Your measurements will improve. Your clothes will be looser. Your physician will be able to measure statistically significant improvements in your cholesterol profile, body fat percentage, inflammatory markers in your blood and most likely your blood pressure. All of these results can be obtained in just five weeks. We've seen it happen over and over with hundreds of our clients, friends and family members. The best part is that your entire family can follow the Gold Coast Cure lifestyle together. The foods we recommend are nutritious *and* delicious, so that you can prepare one meal and satisfy everyone in your household. Everybody, especially growing children, should be eating the balanced, nutrient-rich whole foods we recommend.

The Cure stands out among alternative health and wellness books because our advice is scientifically proven and socially realistic. Our general philosophy is one of moderation and balance. The substitutions are simple, and the additions are painless. Switch from margarine to all-natural, better-tasting spreads. Cook with extra-virgin olive oil instead of standard vegetable oil. Use flax oil and extra-virgin olive oil instead of standard vegetable oils in your salad dressings. Switch from refined, processed grains to whole grains. Use whole-wheat flour products instead of enriched flour products to ensure that you are fueling yourself with nutrients instead of empty carbs. Supplement with essential fats, vitamins and antioxidants. Add omega-3 foods to your diet. Eliminate trans fats from your diet. Perform our resistance circuit-training workout for thirty minutes three times per week. Making even one of these changes can result in markedly improved overall health.

We hope we've provided sufficient motivation. We hope our story and the stories of our clients serve as inspiration. For us it took the diagnosis of multiple sclerosis. What will it take for you to improve your lifestyle?

In today's world, you, not your physician, must be your own advocate. You must take charge of your health, and you must take the initiative to educate yourself. Your doctor can't explain the principles in this book during a ten-minute office visit. We're giving you the opportunity to become your own advocate with the Gold Coast Cure. So make a difference. Take charge like so many of our clients already have. Have fun along the way. You only have one life. Make it a good one.

Part One

Positive Changes Mean Positive Results: Using the Cure to Heal Yourself

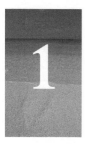

Eliminating the 7 Deadly Dietary Habits

Twenty-first-century medical care is better than ever. We're living longer, doctors have access to the latest medical techniques, and scientists are better able to research and detect disease—yet a glance through the newspaper or a few minutes in front of the TV proves that chronic diseases such as diabetes, cancer, asthma and obesity are on the rise. We can clone animals, create babies through in-vitro fertilization or give someone a new heart, yet our bodies are betraying us, giving in to chronic illnesses that our physicians are powerless to heal.

As far as we've come in the past fifty years, one important aspect of our lives has taken a giant step backward: our diets. Unfortunately, even those of us who think we're health conscious because we buy multigrain cereal or reduced-fat salad dressing may have swapped one bad choice for another, seriously compromising our overall health in the process. We're at the mercy of mass food producers, advertisers and physicians who offer conflicting and sometimes erroneous information. One day we're told the best diet is low fat, and the next day we read we should shun carbs to lose weight and gain health.

All ten of the diseases we target—arthritis, asthma, heart disease, allergies, fibromyalgia, type II diabetes, vascular dementia, obesity, osteoporosis and, of course, multiple sclerosis—are directly related to the foods you eat. Poor food choices—whether you make them intentionally or not—cause increased inflammation and malnutrition, two dietary pariahs that create disease and worsen pre-existing conditions.

The Big "I"— Inflammation

Despite the availability of powerful new medications, inflammatory diseases like fibromyalgia, asthma, allergies, multiple sclerosis, arthritis, psoriasis, heart disease and senility are on the rise in our society. Why? Because our modern diet is far more pro-inflammatory than our ancestors'.

Most of us are so busy trying to keep up with modern life that we eat too many processed convenience foods, many of which are advertised as healthy. Because the human body wasn't designed to process these very refined foods efficiently, if you eat too many of them you set up a chain reaction that causes inflammation in your body. Inflammation contributes to the severity of all of the diseases we target in this book.

The good news is we'll show you how you can control the symptoms of these conditions by reducing the amount of inflammation in your body with an anti-inflammatory diet. As Ivy's success has proven, food is extremely powerful medicine.

The Big "M"— Malnutrition in the Land of Plenty?

While you wouldn't normally think of our society as being malnourished given our seemingly endless supply of cheap, readily available food—and knowing that nearly 65 percent of us are overweight—the truth is that we are not properly nourished. Malnutrition refers to *improper nutrition,* not necessarily inadequate calorie intake. Even though most of us get enough calories to eat, we're often getting these calories in the form of packaged convenience foods from which essential nutrients have been stripped during processing. Therefore, many of us don't consistently get the *nutrients* we need to maintain healthy immune systems, prevent colds and cancer, and ward off obesity. Only natural, whole foods contain all of the important disease-fighting nutrients your body needs.

Many of us further compromise our nutrient intake by trying "food elimination" diets. Chances are, if you've ever been on a low-fat or low-carb diet you were not giving your body the nutrients it needed.

The malnourished body is hungrier than it needs to be and it experiences unnecessary food cravvings; if you are constantly hungry and fighting food cravings then you are at a high risk for obesity and type II diabetes. These conditions are intimely related to not feeling full enough and not being properly nourished. Both conditions can be reversed and prevented following the Cure.

Why Low-Fat Diets Lead to Malnutrition and Inflammation

For years we've been encouraged by well-meaning nutritionists to stuff our grocery carts with fat-free foods to lose weight and enjoy better cardiovascular health. In the past, many of us listened, dutifully munching on fat-free, albeit highly refined, pretzels, bagels, breads and pasta. We were encouraged by the medical community to do this based upon incomplete 1970s-era research that failed to distinguish between healthy fats and unhealthy fats. Because saturated fat is not healthy, *all* fats were assumed to be unhealthy.

At the same time they were missing the boat on fats, doctors failed to properly differentiate between healthy, nutrient-rich carbohydrates and unhealthy, highly processed, nutrient-poor carbohydrates. We were told to eat less sugar but we were never told to avoid the other nutrient-poor carbohydrate—refined flour. In the process, many of us ended up eating hundreds of empty calories a day, setting up a vicious cycle of obesity and other serious health issues. These low-fat advocates failed to remind us that if we didn't immediately burn these empty carbohydrates for energy, then they would be converted into the very thing we were trying to avoid: saturated fat, which blocks our bodies from making many anti-inflammatory hormones, thereby worsening inflammatory diseases.

Why Low-Carb Dieting Leads to Malnutrition and Inflammation

After the low-fat wave came the latest "food-elimination" craze: the low-carb diet fad. Contrary to the low-carb mantra, the truth is that *all* fruits and vegetables are good for you, as are all whole-grain sources of dense carbohydrates, including whole grain breads, whole-grain pasta, beans, legumes and starchy vegetables such as corn, yams and potatoes.

Carbohydrates are the "energy" nutrient, and your body *needs* energy to function. While your body can use fat for energy if it must, it normally only uses fat for energy when it's starving. To protect itself from starving, your body slows down its metabolic rate when you dramatically reduce all carbs, which makes it increasingly difficult for you to lose weight. This decrease in metabolic rate is easily perceived by your brain, which sends out food cravings to signal that it needs carbohydrate energy to meet the stresses of everyday life.

Low-carb diets are far from optimal when it comes to your long-term health, and they lack disease- and obesity-fighting substances such as fiber and phytochemicals. Low-carb dieters almost always over-consume harmful unhealthy fats that dramatically increase inflammation and dramatically worsen diseases mediated by inflammation such as heart disease, multiple sclerosis, asthma and arthritis.

Low-carb dieting leaves you susceptible to health problems in the long run because on this type of "avoidance" diet you consistently fail to obtain optimal amounts of key nutrients your body needs to fight disease.

Low-carbohydrate diets are far from optimal for long-term weight management. One recent study showed the effectiveness of low-carb dieting seems to dwindle over time. In one yearlong *New England Journal of Medicine* study, low-carb dieters ended up gaining enough weight back in the second six months of the study that the difference in weight loss between the low-carb group and the low-fat group was no longer statistically significant by year's end.[1]

The 7 Deadly Dietary Habits

In researching the Gold Coast Cure we've identified the seven deadliest dietary habits. Let's take a look at these habits and see how the Cure eliminates them.

Deadly Habit #1: Eating Too Much Trans Fat

While trans fats have only recently been discussed in the popular wellness literature, the health risks associated with these fats have been known for years. Trans fats are the *absolute worst fats and should not be eaten at all.* Recently, the U.S. National Academy of Science's Institute of Medicine, the organization responsible for advising the U.S. government on health policy and responsible for determining the reference daily intake (RDI) for vitamins, concluded there is absolutely *no safe level of intake* for trans fat.[2] Any food item listing "partially hydrogenated" or "hydrogenated oil" of any type, "margarine," or "vegetable shortening" on its list of ingredients always contains at least some deadly trans fat. Also assume that all fried foods at restaurants and fast-food places contain trans fat. All of these products should be completely avoided.

Trans fats are directly linked with heart disease. Alarmingly, trans fats are capable of altering your cholesterol profile toward the most dangerous ratio in terms of risk for heart disease and are even worse for you than saturated fat. Trans fats raise your bad LDL cholesterol level *and* your total cholesterol level while simultaneously lowering your good protective HDL cholesterol level.[3] If all this isn't bad enough, trans fats also increase your triglyceride level and impair artery dilation, a one-two punch that further increases your risk for heart artery disease.

In a 1993 study in the prestigious medical journal *Lancet*, almost 90,000 healthy women were followed for eight years. There was a 50 percent increase in heart attacks and deaths in those women who ate just 5.7 grams per day of trans fats compared to women who ate only 2.4 grams per day of trans fat. Statistically, this difference was highly significant.[4] The difference between 2.4 and 5.7 grams is less than one order of medium McDonald's french fries or one standard-size glazed donut.

According to evidence reported in 1999 by the Harvard University Department of Nutrition, up to 100,000 premature coronary deaths per year could be prevented by replacing partially hydrogenated oils with natural nonhydrogenated oils.[5] Trans fats have also been linked to conditions other than heart disease. Trans fats block healthy fats from being converted into helpful inflammation fighters and cause your body to produce *more* inflammatory mediators,[6] which increase blood clotting, increase blood pressure and worsen inflammation-mediated conditions such as multiple sclerosis, arthritis, Crohn's disease, psoriasis and asthma.

The Terrible Trans Fat Transformation

Trans fats begin innocently enough as liquid vegetable oil. In their natural, unrefined state *some* of these oils are rich in the healthy fats we'll talk more about later. The problem is that liquid vegetable oil spoils easily. Obviously, high spoilage rates are not economical for cost-sensitive food manufacturers.

Food manufacturers use a chemical process called hydrogenation to extend shelf life and maximize profit. During hydrogenation, the chemical composition of vegetable oil is completely altered. The oils are heated to extremely high temperatures and hydrogen gas is bubbled through them. These extremely high temperatures burn out all of the healthy fats and nutrients while creating toxic free radicals that harm your body.

One of the most important things you can do to improve your health is to avoid all foods containing hydrogenated or partially hydrogenated oil, margarine and vegetable shortening.

THE GOLD COAST CURE SOLUTION: **Eliminate trans fat completely and switch to the healthy alternatives we recommend in chapter 5.**

Deadly Habit #2: Eating Too Many Processed, Nutrient-Poor Carbs and Not Enough Healthy, Whole Carbs

Contrary to popular belief, there are only two carbohydrate foods you need to watch out for: refined flour and sugar. The bad news is the vast majority of the carbohydrate-containing foods the average person eats are made with refined flour and/or sugar. Standard pasta, most breads, most breakfast cereals, pretzels, standard pizza dough, cookies, cakes, most bagels, muffins and standard crackers are all examples of foods that typically contain refined flour, sugar or both.

These two empty-carbohydrate foods—refined flour and sugar—contribute directly to diabetes, obesity, heart disease and a number of inflammatory conditions. The good news is, there are plenty of "whole-carb" alternatives to the empty ones. You can enjoy bread, pasta, cereal and pizza as long as you buy whole-carb products. We'll show you how.

The Big 3: How Empty Carbs Contribute to Obesity, Heart Disease and Diabetes

Obesity and Empty Carbohydrates. Many popular diets advocate that we leave all carbohydrates behind on the path toward weight loss, yet the widely held dietary belief that carbohydrates are always the bad guys is not only incorrect but dangerous in the long term. While fake, empty carbs like white flour bagels, pretzels, white pasta and white bread significantly contribute to obesity, their healthy and nutrient-rich cousins—whole grains, beans, legumes, fruits, vegetables and potatoes—are key in maintaining health and lasting weight loss. Your body needs the nutrients and fiber in healthy, whole-food carbohydrates in order to satisfy food cravings and fight obesity.

Fake, empty carbs are enemy number one when it comes to obesity. When you eat empty carbohydrates, your blood sugar level spikes so your body produces a lot of insulin to bring your blood sugar level back down. The problem is, insulin is your body's principal fat storage hormone; it forces your liver to convert the excess sugar in your blood into fat, then makes your blood deliver this fat to your fat cells, literally packing them with fat. Making a bad situation worse, high circulating levels of insulin prevent your body's fat stores from being used as an energy source. This combination of increased fat storage and decreased fat release con-tributes greatly to obesity. It's a catch-22 that you can stop by avoiding empty carbohydrates.

Poor blood sugar control is another problem closely associated with eat-ing empty carbohydrates. You already know eating empty carbohydrates forces your body to produce a lot of insulin; the problem is, excessive amounts of insulin can drive your blood sugar level too low. When your blood sugar level gets too low you feel hungrier than nature intended for you to be. In other words, you feel hungry even though you don't really need to eat more food. Bad news if you are trying to shed pounds or main-tain your weight.

Heart Disease and Empty Carbohydrates. Although most people blame dietary cholesterol and dietary fat for heart disease, nutrient-poor carbohy-drates are every bit as much to blame for heart problems.

Almost everyone knows saturated fat is bad for the heart. What is less well known is that nutrient-poor carbs are easily converted by your liver into artery-clogging saturated fats if they are eaten in excess of what your body needs for energy. Carbohydrates are the "energy" nutrient, and due to evolution, the human body has become very energy-efficient. There's no reason to keep carbohydrate energy around if you don't use it, so the most efficient thing to do from an evolutionary standpoint is convert these unburned carbohydrates into fat to be stored in your fat cells in case there is a famine. In modern America, this famine never comes, and our waistlines increase. Unless you're so active that your body can immediately use these extra carbohydrates to fuel some sort of activity they *will* be converted into saturated fat.

Eating empty carbohydrates in excess also increases your triglyceride level,[7] which is not good for your cardiovascular health. In fact, some researchers have even suggested that the combination of a high triglyceride level and a low "good" HDL cholesterol level is a more important risk factor for heart disease and stroke than the traditional risk factor of having an increased "bad" LDL cholesterol level.[8]

Even if you ignore the complicating issue of your HDL cholesterol, having an elevated triglyceride level has been proven to be dangerous in and of itself.[9] If you eat fewer overly processed, nutrient-poor carbohydrates you will have fewer triglycerides in your bloodstream, and you will be less likely to develop heart disease.

Diabetes and Empty Carbohydrates. The most common type of diabetes, type II "adult-onset" diabetes, is caused by a malfunction in the way the body handles insulin. Most diabetics start out healthy but eventually become resistant to the effects of their own naturally occurring insulin, leaving their bodies unable to process sugar correctly.

Because processed, empty carbohydrates are a recent human invention, our bodies didn't evolve to handle these foods. Excess intake of empty carbohydrates is the most important preventable cause of insulin resistance.

Empty carbohydrates are digested much more quickly than the fats, proteins and nutrient-rich carbohydrates that your body craves and needs. The rapid digestion of empty carbs causes your blood sugar level to rise rapidly, which triggers your body to release insulin to direct this sugar out of your blood and back into your cells where it can be used for energy. High blood sugar levels equal high insulin levels. If you frequently eat empty carbs, you force your body to produce large amounts of insulin to avoid high blood sugar levels.

Diabetes develops when insulin is produced in such large amounts over such a long period of time that your body eventually becomes resistant to its effect. For a while you get by because your body can produce extra insulin to overcome this resistance. Eventually, though, insulin resistance increases to the point that your body can't produce enough insulin to keep your blood sugar level normal. Now you have diabetes, a powerful risk factor for stroke, heart attack, dementia, amputations, kidney failure, impotence, blindness and more.

In this era of food subtraction, this era of low-fat, low-calorie and low-carbohydrate dieting, the benefits associated with eating whole-foods carbohydrates have been largely overlooked—despite the fact that the whole-foods approach to eating has been shown to be superior to all other dietary lifestyles when it comes to preventing coronary heart disease![10] The difference between a healthful, balanced whole-foods lifestyle and conventional dieting when it comes to heart disease can be greater than 70 percent, far greater than the benefit offered by medications such as aspirin, beta-blockers, cholesterol-lowering drugs or any pills on the market for that matter.

Rather than focusing on subtracting carbs, the Cure emphasizes the importance of striking a healthy balance.

The Cure Diet Is High in Nutrient-Rich, Whole-Foods Carbohydrates

Nutrient rich, whole-foods carbohydrates stabilize your blood sugar level. Nutrient-rich carbs raise your blood sugar level minimally and temporarily. This results in a much less pronounced insulin "spike" than occurs when you eat empty carbohydrates. The more stable your blood sugar level, the less likely you are to become hungry and the easier it is for you to lose weight and maintain your weight. Also, the more stable your blood sugar level, the less likely you are to become insulin resistant and diabetic.

Once you learn to balance your blood sugar level by consistently eating whole-foods carbohydrates, your appetite will naturally fall within a normal range. Eating unprocessed whole-foods carbohydrates allows you, not your blood sugar level, to be in control of your appetite.

THE GOLD COAST CURE SOLUTION: **Eat balanced meals containing nutrient-rich whole carbs such as whole wheat pasta, whole grain bread, potatoes, brown rice, oatmeal, beans, fruits and vegetables.**

Deadly Habit #3: Eating Too Much Saturated Fat

Doctors and nutritionists have been giving the public sound advice in the saturated fat department for at least thirty years. By now most of us know that if we eat too much saturated fat (the fat found in butter, high-fat dairy foods, fatty meats and some processed foods), we increase our risk of heart attack, high cholesterol, stroke and peripheral vascular disease. Less publicized is that diets rich in saturated fat also contribute to gallbladder disease[11] and certain types of cancer, as well as fibromyalgia, multiple sclerosis,[12] asthma,[13] vascular dementia, allergies, arthritis and psoriasis. Saturated fats interfere with the way your body regulates its production of natural hormones called prostaglandins, the hormones that fight inflammation in your body.

THE GOLD COAST CURE SOLUTION: **Healthy people should limit their saturated fat intake to 20 grams per day; people with heart conditions or other inflammatory conditions should limit saturated fat to 15 grams per day. This is the *only* counting you need to do on the Cure.**
Don't worry; sticking to our saturated fat budget is not difficult. You are still allowed to eat foods containing saturated fat in moderation, and there are many other healthful fats you can enjoy in large quantity instead.

Deadly Habit #4: Not Eating Enough Essential Fat

There are two types of healthy essential fat: omega-3 fat and omega-6 fat. Your body needs these good fats on a steady basis to rebuild cells;

support brain function; burn fat stores for fuel; maintain the health of your cardiovascular, reproductive, central nervous and immune systems; and much more. Every living cell in your body either directly or indirectly needs essential fats in order to function properly. Modern diets are more deficient in the highly anti-inflammatory omega-3 essential fat than they are in any other type of food.

When people hear the word "fat," they get scared, yet essential fats actually assist with weight loss. Essential fats are highly unsaturated fats that burn faster than other fats. They have the unique ability to *increase* your metabolic rate, forcing your body to burn excess body fat. In his bestselling book, *Fats That Heal, Fats That Kill,* Udo Erasmus explains, "In these (high) quantities, EFA's (essential fatty acids) help burn off excess fats, and help a person to lose weight and stay slim."[14] A study from the Netherlands confirms that diets high in polyunsaturated (essential) fat increase your resting metabolic rate by almost 4 percent when compared against diets high in saturated fat.[15] This adds up to about fifty extra calories burned per day. That's over five pounds per year, even if you consume the same amount of food, and even if you just sit still!

Unlike other fats, essential fats are not used by your body for energy unless all other calorie sources are completely exhausted. Therefore, essential fats are not stored as body fat. Instead, they're used for the continuous maintenance of critical structural, hormonal and electrical functions within your body.

Because essential fats nourish your skin, an essential fat deficiency can lead to brittle hair, weak nails, a bad complexion and premature skin aging. You absolutely cannot achieve an optimally beautiful complexion from creams alone. Dermatologists know essential fats promote health and vitality from the inside out. Acne-prone patients are often encouraged by cutting-edge dermatologists to supplement their diets with essential fats while eliminating or drastically reducing foods rich in saturated fat and trans fats. Interestingly, acne is a rare condition in cultures where whole-food diets predominate.[16]

Mature skin benefits as well because essential fats allow your skin to retain moisture, helping to ward off the dreaded "prune" face. Men and women on wrinkle patrol should become more aware of the crucial role essential fats play in keeping the complexion smooth, supple and moisturized. Los Angeles plastic surgeon Richard Ellenbogen states ". . . very low fat diets suck the oils out of our skin. We see people in their thirties on low fat diets who look like prunes. . . ."[17]

Eating more essential fats provides numerous specific health benefits. Below, we highlight just some of the scientifically proven health benefits.

Table 1.1
Health Benefits Associated with
Essential Fat Consumption

1. Decreased risk of stroke and heart attack
2. Significantly reduced triglyceride levels
3. Reduced blood pressure
4. Protection against many types of cancer
5. Reduced severity of depression symptoms
6. Protection against:
   - Multiple sclerosis
   - Arthritis
   - Crohn's disease
   - Asthma
   - Ulcerative colitis
   - Vascular dementia
   - Dysmenorrhea (menstrual pain)
   - Psoriasis
   - Fibromyalgia
   - Allergies
7. Improved resistance to infection
8. Reduced risk of developing osteoporosis.[18, 19]

THE GOLD COAST CURE SOLUTION: **The Cure Is High in Anti-Inflammatory Essential Fats.** You will increase your overall intake of essential fat by eating whole-food sources of omega-6 essential fat such as soybeans, whole grains and nuts. You'll learn how to easily incorporate omega-3 fats into your diet by eating foods such as fish, shellfish, walnuts, expeller-pressed canola oil, flaxseeds and flax oil more frequently.

Deadly Habit #5: Eating Too Much Processed Vegetable Oil

Saturated fat was identified as a risk factor for heart disease nearly forty years ago. Consequently, health-conscious individuals began to limit their intake of saturated fat and food manufacturers jumped on the bandwagon, reducing the saturated fat content of foods by replacing it with processed vegetable oils. Today, vegetable oils are used in excess quantities in an enormous amount of processed foods. Look around and you'll find a very large percentage of prepackaged, processed foods contain either some sort of vegetable oil or some sort of partially hydrogenated vegetable oil.

Mass-market vegetable oils are refined at very high temperatures, processed, made rancid so they last longer, then deodorized and purified to make their taste "acceptable." These grocery-store-quality vegetable oils are empty calorie foods that damage your health and expand your waistline.

Despite their healthy sounding name, standard vegetable oils can be *very harmful* to your overall health. These oils include standard sunflower oil, standard safflower oil, corn oil, sesame oil, peanut oil, soybean oil, cottonseed oil and "pure" vegetable oil.

Why Are Processed Vegetable Oils So Bad for You?

There are three crucial reasons we consider mass-market vegetable oils to be damaging to your health:

Standard vegetable oils are processed improperly. Vegetable oils consist primarily of essential but highly perishable omega-6 fats. While omega-6 fats are healthy in their natural unadulterated state, they're harmful when they're processed and handled improperly. Omega-6 fats must be protected from heat, light and air, otherwise they become damaged, unhealthful fats. The standard highly refined vegetable oils we listed above are usually not processed properly because it's very expensive to do so. The vast majority of grocery stores can't afford to stock high-quality vegetable oils, and so for the most part they don't.

Vegetable oil is an empty calorie food. Grocery store vegetable oils are made from healthy "whole foods" such as corn, soybeans and peanuts. The problem is modern-day processing techniques remove all of the nutrients and all of the fiber from these whole foods. The end product, processed vegetable oil, is nutrient poor and calorie rich.

Vegetable oil has the wrong omega-3 to omega-6 ratio. When it comes to essential fat, we need more omega-3 fat but not necessarily more omega-6 fat. The average person eats a very unbalanced ratio of omega-3 essential fat to omega-6 essential fat. As a society, over the last few decades we've dramatically increased our intake of highly refined, omega-6 fat-rich vegetable oils. As a result, we now eat *too much* refined omega-6 fat and *too little* omega-3 fat, the type of fat found mostly in fish, shellfish, walnuts, expeller-pressed canola oil, flax seeds and flax oil.

In order to control inflammatory diseases you should consume no more than about four times more omega-6 fat than omega-3 fat. The average person on the typical modern diet eats approximately fourteen to twenty times more omega-6 fat than omega-3 fat!

Why Is the Omega Ratio So Important?

Eating the correct ratio of omega-3 fat to omega-6 fat maximizes your production of good anti-inflammatory prostaglandins while reducing your production of bad pro-inflammatory prostaglandins. If omega-6 fats are eaten in reasonable amounts, they are converted almost exclusively into good anti-inflammatory prostaglandins. However, when omega-6 fats are eaten in excess they can be converted into substances your body later uses to make bad pro-inflammatory prostaglandins. *Pro-inflammatory prostaglandins worsen any disease mediated by inflammation.*

It's not hard to change your diet to optimize your omega ratio. If you eliminate only a few harmful vegetable oils from your diet and simultaneously increase your intake of the good omega-3 fats we recommend later, you're all set. No calculating. No thinking. It really is that simple.

Although the public in general is unaware of the significance the omega ratio has on overall health and well-being, established medical and nutritional journals have repeatedly reported on the benefits derived from eating the correct essential fat ratio. Unbalanced essential fat intake has been linked to various serious degenerative conditions including heart disease, several cancers, stroke, asthma, rheumatoid arthritis and vascular dementia.[20]

THE GOLD COAST CURE SOLUTION: **Switch from deadly mass-market oils to properly prepared, unheated omega-3 oils,** such as flax oil and expeller-pressed canola oil, and other healthful oils such as extra-virgin olive oil, avocado oil and the special high-oleic versions of sunflower, safflower and canola oils that are now for sale. Plenty of healthful oils exist, and plenty of healthful oils are allowed on the Gold Coast Cure.

Deadly Habit #6: Not Eating Enough Fiber

Fiber is found in nutrient-rich carbohydrate foods such as beans, whole-grain bread, whole-grain pasta, potatoes, brown rice, corn, peas, fruits and vegetables—many foods that are shunned by those on low-carb diets. Fiber is not found in overly processed, refined carbohydrates such as white pasta, breads made using refined flour, white rice and standard pizza dough.

Fiber has numerous proven, significant health benefits, and fiber is a trusted ally when it comes to weight management. Fiber deficiency largely explains the twin pandemics of diabetes and obesity. Consider the following fiber facts:

- Fiber decreases your risk of developing colon and rectal cancer by as much as 50 percent.[21] Fiber prevents other intestinal diseases including diverticulosis and diverticulitis, potentially lethal diseases of the colon. In countries where high fiber diets are eaten, diverticulosis and diverticulitis are very rare. Studies suggest that about half of all symptomatic cases of these diseases would be prevented by adhering to a higher fiber diet.[22]
- Fiber is nature's detoxifier, helping to remove nondigestible toxins from your body.
- Fiber improves your cholesterol profile.
- Fiber slows down digestion of all the foods you eat and consequently helps stabilize your blood sugar level. This means less diabetes, less obesity and less hunger.
- Fiber helps you lose weight. Researchers at Tufts University have shown that people who add an additional 14 grams of fiber to their daily diet end up eating 10 percent fewer calories when all is said and done.[23] In another study, university researchers in Ontario used detailed food diaries to compare the total daily fiber intake of cross sections of the Canadian public.[24] The people in this study who maintained a healthy weight were eating 30 percent more fiber than those who were overweight.

THE GOLD COAST CURE SOLUTION: **By following the Gold Coast Cure, you can effortlessly double or even triple your current fiber intake.**

Deadly Habit #7: Not Eating Enough Micronutrients

Fats, proteins and carbohydrates are collectively referred to as macronutrients, and vitamins, minerals, antioxidants and phyto-chemicals are collectively referred to as *micro*nutrients.

Modern diets are deficient in micronutrients. It's true that modern foods are fortified with vitamins and minerals. For this reason most of us are neither vitamin nor mineral deficient. The problem is that processed foods are not fortified with all of the other antioxidants and phytochemicals that are present in natural, whole foods. These substances are destroyed by processing, and they are rarely, if ever, replaced.

Unlike vitamins and minerals, antioxidants and phytochemicals are not absolutely essential for life itself. Nevertheless, these naturally occurring substances are essential if you want to enjoy optimal health. Antioxidants and phytochemicals provide protection against heart disease, dementia, stroke, autoimmune diseases, cataracts, certain cancers and many other conditions. Antioxidants are anti-aging "super nutrients" that work around the clock to protect your body from environmental pollution. Phytochemicals are healthful substances found only in carbohydrate-containing plant-based foods. Scientific evidence supports the value of phytochemicals in preventing and treating at least three leading causes of premature death, namely cancer,[25] hypertension and cardiovascular disease. Only natural, whole foods contain all the micronutrients you need for optimal health.

THE GOLD COAST CURE SOLUTION: **Eat a wide variety of whole foods to obtain optimal amounts of micronutrients.**

Now you know the basic concepts of the Cure. In the next few chapters, we'll walk you through how to make healthful food choices that heal your body and slim your waistline. If you're ready to put the Cure to work for you right away, feel free to skip ahead to chapter 8 where you'll learn how to outfit a Gold Coast Cure kitchen so you can start enjoying the delicious Gold Coast Cure meal plans.

Avoiding the Empty Carbs That Make You Fat and Sick

As we noted in the last chapter, calorie for calorie, empty carbohydrates are the foods most likely to increase your risk for heart disease and diabetes. Empty carbs also contribute to weight gain and obesity. These foods are extremely easy to overeat because they are devoid of fiber, and when overeaten, empty carbs are converted into saturated fats, which increase inflammation. In this chapter we'll give you the tools you need to avoid these dangerous carbs.

Empty Carb #1: Refined Flour

The typical American likes to eat pizza, pasta, doughnuts and cookies. Even when we think we're being "good" by choosing wheat bread because it's low in fat, or crackers that seem "healthy," the majority of these foods are made from refined flour and therefore they are not healthy.

While the vast majority of flour sold in Western countries is made from wheat, the nutrient-rich wheat germ and the fiber-rich wheat bran are removed during processing, leaving only the nutrient-poor, fiber-free starch. *No nutrients equals empty calories.* Rapidly absorbed nutrient-poor carbs lead to weight gain, insulin resistance, hunger, obesity, diabetes, heart disease and, indirectly, to a host of inflammatory conditions.

The Whole Truth

"Whole" wheat flours, and all other "whole" grain flours, are healthful carbohydrates because they're made from the entire grain kernel. For example, whole-wheat flour contains the wheat germ (full of nutrients) and the ground-up wheat bran (lots of fiber) in addition to the wheat starch (calorie energy). Because nothing is removed, whole-grain flours are rich in fiber, vitamins, minerals and antioxidants. There are plenty of healthful products out there made with whole-wheat flour and other whole-grain flours, so you need *not* banish baked goods while following the Cure.

Translating Labels

Very few food product labels use the term "refined" flour in their listing of ingredients because most manufacturers don't want to draw attention to the fact that their product was refined. For this reason, most food processing firms prefer to use the word "enriched" instead of word "refined." Although enriched flour certainly sounds healthier than refined flour, it isn't. Enrichment refers to the government-mandated process of adding small amounts of synthetic vitamins and minerals to refined flour after it has been processed. As required by law, all refined flour is enriched.

Enriched flour does *not* contain fiber, and the synthetic vitamins that are added represent only a small portion of the nutrients that were removed during processing. Disease-fighting phytochemicals are lost forever during the refinement process and are not added back. In their attempts to pass fake foods off as healthful, food manufacturers may choose to dye refined-flour breads a brownish color by using dyes or adding sugar syrups or molasses to the bread. Obviously, adding brown food dye or molasses does not transform white bread into a health food!

Food manufacturers especially like to splash the word "wheat" on their products because some people erroneously believe wheat bread and other wheat products are somehow more healthful than white products. The food processing companies are not lying. Yes, indeed, the bread was made from wheat. Even white bread starts out as healthy wheat kernels.

Manufacturers also love the word "multigrain." Many multigrain products contain only enriched, refined versions of more than one grain. The typical multigrain product is no more healthful than white bread. While it's great to eat grains other than just wheat—because variety assures you are exposed to more of the phytochemicals, antioxidants and micronutrients nature has to offer—this approach only works if you eat *whole grains*.

Processed Foods to Avoid

The list of foods in Table 2.1 is long because most commercial preparations do not use whole grains. It's definitely possible to find or make breads, rolls, cakes and so on from whole grains. In our "Kitchen Shape-Up" (chapter 8), we'll show you how to locate more healthful, better-tasting versions of just about every refined flour carbohydrate food appearing on this table.

The products listed in Table 2.1 are almost always made from refined or enriched flours unless the labeling specifically states other-wise. Always read the list of ingredients before buying these foods.

BOTTOM LINE ———————————————————————

Avoid foods made with refined flour.

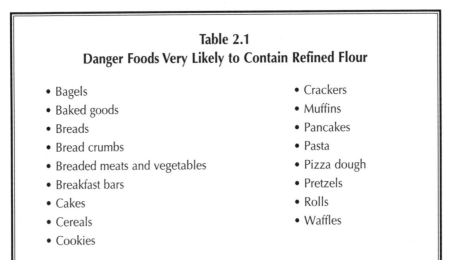

Table 2.1
Danger Foods Very Likely to Contain Refined Flour

- Bagels
- Baked goods
- Breads
- Bread crumbs
- Breaded meats and vegetables
- Breakfast bars
- Cakes
- Cereals
- Cookies
- Crackers
- Muffins
- Pancakes
- Pasta
- Pizza dough
- Pretzels
- Rolls
- Waffles

Empty Carb #2: Sugar

Almost any five-year-old can tell you eating too many sweets is not healthy. No loving mother has ever said, "Come on, Johnny, eat your four tablespoons of sugar so you can grow up big, healthy and strong." Little Johnny might grow up big—too big—on a high sugar diet, but he won't grow up healthy.

Why is sugar so unhealthful? Sugar supplies a quick source of energy, but it contains no other useful nutrients. You are much better off eating nutrient-rich carbohydrates that contain energy plus nutrients and fiber as opposed to empty-calorie carbs that provide energy but no nutrition. This having been said, we believe it's important to enjoy our meals, so we do allow some exceptions to the sugar rule, which we will discuss just a little bit later. Sugar lovers may rest assured that the Cure lifestyle does allow for some "cheating."

According to the United States Department of Agriculture, the average U.S. resident eats more than sixty-four pounds of sugar every year! To put that into perspective, sixty-four pounds of sugar translates into a whopping 108,800 empty calories eaten per person per year. If the

Strategic Shopping: The Rules
for Finding Healthful Packaged Foods

Always look for the word "whole" in the list of ingredients. Be suspicious of breads and other carbohydrate-based foods advertised as being "made from whole wheat" or "made with whole grains" because current labeling regulations allow manufacturers to use the words "whole grain" on the packaging as long as 51 percent of the product by weight is whole grain. Given this little problem, what should you do? Here are two solid strategies:

1. The first strategy is to look for the first item on the list of ingredients. The first ingredient *must* be either a whole food such as oatmeal, brown rice, corn or whole wheat kernels or, if the first ingredient is "flour," the word "whole" must appear before the word "flour." Look for the words "whole wheat flour" instead of "wheat flour," for example. If the first ingredient is a whole food, then the food is probably acceptable even if a few other ingredients listed further down are not quite so healthy. We don't live in a perfect world.

2. The second strategy is to look at both the fiber content per serving and the total number of carbohydrate grams per serving. This information is required by law to be on the label. In any carbohydrate-based food there should always be *at the very least 2 grams of fiber per 25 grams of carbohydrate.* Three grams of fiber or more per 25 grams of carbohydrate is even better, especially if you are diabetic, overweight or trying to lose weight. More fiber is always better.

These two simple rules put you in charge of your health at the grocery store. They apply to all packaged carbohydrate-based foods. You don't have to apply these rules to fruits, vegetables and other products that are not packaged.

average person cut his or her sugar consumption down by just two-thirds, he or she could lose up to twenty pounds in one year!

While most of us accurately report enjoying desserts and added sugar in moderation, we still consume an unhealthy 30 percent of our total daily carbohydrate intake in the form of added sugar. This is primarily because sugar "proxies" lurk amongst the ingredients in a huge assortment of packaged, processed foods. If you eat a diet rich in packaged foods, you are almost positively eating far more sugar than you think you are.

Start reading labels and you'll find sugar is hidden in everything from spaghetti sauces to breakfast cereals to frozen food entrées. But sugar is rarely called "sugar" on the ingredient list; it goes by many aliases. You need to watch out for added, non-natural sugars, so read labels carefully. Table 2.2 lists some of the most common sugar pseudonyms.

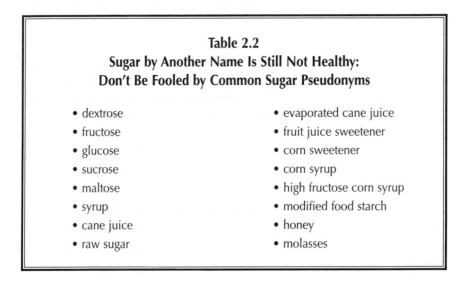

Table 2.2
Sugar by Another Name Is Still Not Healthy:
Don't Be Fooled by Common Sugar Pseudonyms

• dextrose	• evaporated cane juice
• fructose	• fruit juice sweetener
• glucose	• corn sweetener
• sucrose	• corn syrup
• maltose	• high fructose corn syrup
• syrup	• modified food starch
• cane juice	• honey
• raw sugar	• molasses

The "Least Bad" Sugars to Eat in Moderation

Although we classify all sugars as nutrient-poor, empty carbohydrates, some sugars are worse than others when it comes to your health. The least bad sugars are less refined, and they do contain some nutrients as compared with the worst offenders. The sugars below are listed in order from most healthful to least healthful. *All* sugars must be eaten in moderation, however, no matter where they happen to appear on this list. (See page 120 for a definition of moderation and how to "cheat" with a daily sweet treat.)

- **Molasses.** Molasses is the very sweet juice obtained from the sugarcane plant. It contains some nutrients, minerals leached from the soil and phytochemicals.
- **Blackstrap Molasses** has had most of the sugar removed and is not particularly sweet, but it's rich in iron and contains some other nutrients.
- **Raw Sugar.** Most raw sugar is obtained from the evaporation of cane juice. In other words, raw sugar is concentrated molasses. Because raw sugar is not refined, it retains some of the nutrients found in the naturally growing sugarcane. Always choose slightly brown raw sugar over refined white sugar. Many health food store products and many all-natural packaged foods use the term "evaporated cane juice" in their labeling. Evaporated cane juice is the same thing as raw sugar.
- **Honey.** Raw honey is a combination of four sugars. It contains some essential nutrients, including several B vitamins, the vitamins C, D, and E, and natural antioxidants.
- **Real Maple Syrup.** While real maple syrup is not nutrient-rich, at least it's all-natural. Avoid fake "maple-flavored" syrups because they often contain artificial colorings, preservatives and loads of corn syrup, a truly bad sugar.

- **Fructose.** Fructose is the natural sugar found in fruit. Although fruits are healthful, fructose alone is not so good. Fructose contains none of the nutrients, none of the antioxidants and none of the fiber found in the whole fruit. Fructose, when not surrounded by the rest of the fruit, is an empty calorie.

  Fructose has one advantage over other sugars. Because it's metabolized in a completely different way than all other sugars, it doesn't cause your insulin level to "spike" and therefore doesn't cause the rapid rise in your blood sugar level that is associated with all other sugars. In theory, this should result in less hunger, less obesity and less diabetes compared with other sugars. In practice this has not been proven. Avoid eating fructose unless you're eating it as part of the whole fruit.

The Truly Bad Sugars to Avoid

The following sugars are all completely refined, contain zero nutrients and only empty calories. These foods should be avoided completely if at all possible. We've put these foods in order from least bad to the absolute worst.

- **Sucrose.** This is the same thing as white, refined table sugar. Sucrose is a combination of glucose and fructose and contains no nutrients.
- **High Fructose Corn Syrup.** Glucose mixed with fructose. Despite being called "high fructose," this product contains about the same amount of fructose as sucrose. High fructose corn syrup is much more heavily processed than table sugar. More chemicals touch the product en route to your plate as compared with sucrose. It contains absolutely no nutrients.
- **Corn Syrup.** This is pure glucose, the worst type of sugar.
- **Corn Sweetener.** Pure glucose.

- **Maltose.** Pure glucose.
- **Modified Food Starch.** This is a bunch of glucose molecules connected to each other; in other words, pure glucose.
- **Dextrose.** Just another name for glucose.
- **Glucose.** This is the simplest, most rapidly digested sugar. No other substance spikes your insulin level faster. Pure glucose is rarely added to food products because it's not as sweet tasting as products such as high fructose corn syrup.

Gold Coast–Approved Treats

No lifestyle can work if it's impossible to follow. We know sweets are a weakness for many of us, so the Cure allows you four specific ways to indulge without compromising optimal health.

1) **A Daily Sweet Treat.** You can enjoy one *small* dessert serving of one unhealthful carbohydrate food every day as long as it is *all natural.* "All natural" is the watchword. Your sweet treat may contain refined flour and sugar. Examples might include a small scoop of ice cream, a cookie or even white bread. Remember, white bread has the same nutritional value as a dessert. *This treat may not contain any hydrogenated oil, partially hydrogenated oil, margarine or vegetable shortening.*

   It is especially important to be mindful of portion size. If you're trying to lose weight, the smaller you make this treat, the faster the weight will come off. As a general rule of thumb, rich desserts such as cheesecake, crème brûlée, a brownie, pie or cake should be no thicker than about 1 inch and no larger than half the size of your palm. Servings of ice cream, puddings, mousse and soufflè should be no larger than 4 ounces, half a cup. Lighter desserts such as apple crisp that contain only a minimal amount of fat or cream and are made primarily with fruit, flour and sugar can be about 1 inch thick and up to the size of your palm but no more!

2) **Chocolate.** Chocolate is not as bad for you as you might think. Although we're not suggesting you make a meal out of Belgian chocolates, a little chocolate now and then is not so bad. In fact, it may even be healthful.

The cocoa bean from which chocolate is made contains disease-fighting phytochemicals and antioxidants. Studies show chocolate can thin your blood and provide protection against heart attacks, vascular senility and the most common type of stroke.[1] Studies show cocoa has more antioxidant power than black tea, green tea or even red wine.[2]

When selecting chocolate, don't settle for anything less than the best. Cheap mass-market milk chocolate candy bars contain deadly trans fats, lots of truly bad refined sugar, and, surprise, almost *no* real chocolate. The chocolate, specifically the cocoa, is the healthful part! Go for gourmet chocolate: the darker the chocolate, the healthier it is for you. Gourmet dark chocolate (such as Godiva) contains more chocolate, less sugar, fewer chemicals, and no hydrogenated or partially hydrogenated oils.

Portion size should be mentioned here, too. We're not recommending that you eat an entire candy bar. Keep your chocolate treats down to about *1 square inch.*

3) **Condiments.** A little bit of sugar is not going to kill you, especially if the food you're eating is otherwise healthful and you eat it in small quantities. By definition, condiments are eaten in small quantities. Many of the most common condiments, such as all-natural ketchups and steak sauces, contain healthful ingredients such as tomatoes, herbs and spices in addition to their not-so-healthy refined sugar.

It is also marginally acceptable to use raw sugar as a condiment in small quantities. Although you shouldn't add heaping tablespoons of sugar to your foods and beverages, it's acceptable to use a little bit of sugar for sweetness as part of a recipe now and then. Eliminate packaged food products that contain sugar as opposed to lightly used condiments.

4) **Sugar Substitutes:** A sugar lover's dream does exist: a product called sucralose that's sold under the trade name Splenda. Splenda is made from sugar yet contains zero calories, zero saccharin and zero aspartame. Most important, it tastes just like sugar. Unlike any other sugar substitute we've tried, Splenda has absolutely no aftertaste. You can substitute Splenda for sugar in any recipe, and it even stands up to high-heat cooking and baking.

If you don't care to use Splenda, stevia is another natural, healthful, noncaloric sweetener that is every bit as safe as Splenda. An herb native to South America, it is extremely sweet and can be purchased at the natural foods store.

Cooking with Splenda

To maintain the most natural taste and consistency possible we recommend you modify sugar-sweetened recipes by using Splenda "Sugar Blend for Baking." This product is part Splenda, part sugar. Just a half-cup of Splenda "Sugar Blend for Baking" replaces a full cup of pure sugar; you will cut your sugar calories in half without sacrificing flavor.

Avoiding Empty Carbs in the Grocery Aisle

The following packaged products are very likely to be nutrient-poor empty-carbohydrate foods unless you make the special effort to purchase healthful versions (please refer to chapter 4 for healthful alternatives).

- **Baked Goods.** Assume all grocery store baked goods products are bad for you. These foods are almost universally made from refined flour. You don't even need to look at the list of ingredients. All breads are unhealthy unless the bread is made primarily from whole grains and other all-natural ingredients. *Use our 2 grams of fiber per 25 grams of carbohydrate rule as an absolute minimum for the fiber content. Three grams of fiber per 25 grams of carbohydrate is always better. Any baked good product listing hydrogenated oil, partially hydrogenated oil or vegetable shortening in its list of ingredients must be avoided completely* no matter how much fiber there is. Croissants and deli-style bagels made with refined flour are always unhealthy.

- **Cereal.** About 85 percent of supermarket cereals are junk. Unfortunately, many well-meaning parents send their kids off to school every morning after a breakfast of junk. Don't rely on misleading advertising claims. Ignore the number of grains found in the cereal, ignore the vitamin content, and ignore the words "fruit," "nut," "healthy," "100 percent" and "enriched." Most supermarket cereals contain a slew of unhealthful ingredients such as sugar, corn syrup, modified food starch and even cheap, processed vegetable oils. Processed cereals are rarely made from whole grains, and most are nearly devoid of fiber.

  Remember the rule of thumb we provided earlier but be even stricter in selecting cereal. If any cereal contains less than 3 grams of fiber per 25 grams of carbohydrate it is an overly processed, bad carbohydrate food. Fiber content is always provided to you on the label by law. All-natural cereal should contain lots of fiber. Many of the healthful cereal brands we recommend in chapter 8 contain 5 or more grams of fiber per serving.

• **Pasta.** Avoid most grocery store pasta and the pasta served at restaurants. However, you do not need to give up pasta entirely: Simply switch to whole-wheat pasta. Whole-wheat pasta is healthful, nutrient-rich, fiber-rich and delicious. Not too long ago you could only find whole-wheat pasta at natural foods stores, but today whole-wheat pasta is available in supermarkets across the country. *Whole-grain pasta contains about 2½ to 3 grams of fiber per 25 grams of carbohydrate.* For those of you who claim you won't like the taste of whole-wheat pasta, try some of the recipes in chapter 14 and 16—you'll soon change your mind.

• **Cookies, Cakes and Sweets.** Almost every commercially prepared cookie, cake and "sweet treat" is unhealthy. Most commercially prepared desserts are made from unnatural ingredients and most include at least some deadly trans fats. Even if they don't contain trans fat, they almost always contain refined vegetable oil, which is nearly as bad. But don't worry, more healthful versions of these treats do exist (please see chapter 8, "Kitchen Shape-Up," for name brands).

• **Crackers.** It's easy to distinguish between the good and the bad because what makes breads and baked goods bad also makes crackers bad. Stick with whole-grain crackers containing 2 or more grams of fiber per 25 grams of carbohydrate. Never eat crackers containing hydrogenated oil, vegetable shortening or refined flour.

• **Muffins.** This is getting easier by now, we hope. You already know breads made with refined flour, loads of sugar and trans fats are not healthy. Ditto for muffins. The same ingredients that make breads, crackers and sweet treats unhealthful also make muffins unhealthful.

When talking about muffins, we really have to mention portion size. Surely you have noticed how the average muffin seems to have grown in size over the past few years. Let's clear up any misconceptions. A single muffin serving is not half the size of your head. A muffin should be the size of a standard muffin cup, no larger.

Carefully read the ingredient label and the fiber content on all prepackaged muffins. *If you buy premade muffins, make sure they're made with whole wheat-flour or some other whole-grain flour and make sure they contain at least 2 to 3 grams of fiber per 25 grams of carbohydrate.* And absolutely no hydrogenated oils!

A common marketing trick used by muffin makers is to call brown-colored muffins "bran" muffins. In almost every case these "bran" muffins are the nutritional equivalent of cake. Made from refined flour, globs of sugar and deadly trans fats, these muffins often contain no bran at all. The word "bran" is obviously not regulated properly.

What's the solution if you're a muffin lover? Either buy your muffins at the natural foods store or make your own (see chapter 12 for recipe ideas).

• **Waffles and Pancakes.** You shouldn't need too much help with this one, either. You already know to avoid products containing hydrogenated and partially hydrogenated oils. You also know you should eat no more than one serving per day of any food made from refined flour and you know too much sugar is not healthful either. *You also know that the fiber content should be at least 2 to 3 grams per 25 grams of carbohydrate.*

Tasty, all-natural, nutrient-rich waffle and pancake mixes are available at your local natural foods store, and some super-markets even carry these more healthful mixes. In the Kitchen Shape-Up chapter we mention Arrowhead Mills and Hodgson Mills as being two quality brand names to look for when selecting healthy pancake and waffle mixes. We also mention healthful frozen waffles, too.

Now that you've gotten the lowdown on the empty carbs to avoid, the next chapter weeds out the harmful fats and oils.

3

Avoiding the Deadly Fats

The Deadliest Fat

Trans fats are used to extend a food's shelf life, but they are proven to decrease human life. Foods containing trans fat are *much more damaging* to your health than foods containing either saturated fat or cholesterol, yet the average health-conscious consumer still fears saturated fats and cholesterol more than trans fat. Don't be fooled. Avoid trans fat at all cost because there is no safe level of intake.

Once you become trans fat savvy, it seems like they lurk everywhere, especially in processed foods. Because trans fats contain no cholesterol you'll often find them in processed foods advertised as "cholesterol free," despite the fact that consumption of trans fats is guaranteed to negatively affect your blood cholesterol profile (even though the effect of eating cholesterol itself is negligible). Trans fats are found in traditional junk foods (such as cakes, doughnuts, potato chips, French fries and cookies), but they're also in foods you may think are healthy, some of which you may give to your children. Don't!

Beware of These Trans Fats Food Traps

Here are just a few examples of seemingly healthful foods that often contain trans fats:

- Breads
- Breakfast cereals
- Cereal bars
- Crackers
- Granola bars
- Fig Newtons
- Many energy or nutrition bars
- Muffins
- Soups
- Frozen "diet" meals

You'll find trans fat in almost all fried foods at any restaurant, fast food or full service, unless specifically stated otherwise in writing. We suggest you do not eat any fried food when eating out. When shopping, if you see *anywhere* on the ingredient list the words "hydrogenated oil," "partially hydrogenated oil," "margarine" or "vegetable shortening" you automatically know the food contains trans fat. Don't eat these foods.

Even more troublesome, some unhealthful food products are now claiming to be "trans fat free" despite containing partially hydrogenated oil or vegetable shortening. Under current law, foods containing less than ½ gram of trans fat are allowed to make this claim. This is absolutely unacceptable from a health standpoint because it takes *very little* trans fat to increase inflammation in your body, reduce your production of good inflammatory fighters and alter your cholesterol profile in a negative way. *Any amount of trans fat is too much.* Always read the list of ingredients. Eliminating trans fats from your diet is one of the simplest lifestyle changes you can make, and it will go very far toward improving your overall health.

There are two foods so laden with trans fat and so commonly eaten we must discuss them individually here. These foods should not be eaten in any quantity, ever. Eliminating just these two foods from your diet will do wonders for your health.

Trans Fat Labeling Laws

As early as May 1994, Harvard School of Public Health researchers, recognizing the ongoing danger to the public, asked the government to mandate placement of trans fat content on food labels and to work with the food industry to substantially decrease the use of partially hydrogenated vegetable oils.[1] Unfortunately, the wheels of progress turn very slowly and only now are these recommendations beginning to be implemented.

At press time, food labeling laws are just barely catching up with the science. The U.S. government is working toward mandating that trans fat content appears on every nutrition label. At this writing, "D-Day" is January 1, 2006. Until then it is your job to be an educated consumer.

Margarine

This little bucket of yellow goop represents one of the biggest health fallacies in the recent past. Advertised as a saturated fat- and cholesterol-free "heart healthy" alternative to butter, this fake food outsells butter to this day, despite the fact that science has proved it to be much worse for your health!

Some physicians have not kept up with the growing body of literature on this subject, and some doctors still tell their patients to make the switch from butter to margarine. Although for a brief period of time it was believed margarine was more healthful than butter, researchers now know otherwise. Margarine does not promote heart health—quite the opposite! Eating margarine in any quantity increases your risk of heart disease. Attorneys searching for the next RJ Reynolds need only look as far as the margarine industry to earn their next billion.

Margarine has been implicated as a leading causative factor in heart attack and death since the early 1990s.[2] In one study, the risk of having a first heart attack was two and a half times greater when comparing people who ate high levels of trans fat to those who ate little trans fat.

There is absolutely no reason to use margarine. The truly heart-healthy spreads, like Smart Balance, available at all major supermarkets, and Earth Balance, available mostly at natural foods stores, contain less than half as much saturated fat as butter, absolutely no trans fats and absolutely no hydrogenated oils. These products rival butter in the taste department and beat the taste of margarine hands down.

Vegetable Shortening

Vegetable shortening is a definite red light! This horribly unhealthful product is one of the most highly hydrogenated products on the market. The word "vegetable" misleads consumers into thinking this garbage is a healthy alternative to butter. Not so!

Read labels carefully because vegetable shortening hides out as an ingredient in numerous grocery products, including the majority of packaged baked goods. Just because you don't add vegetable shortening when you cook doesn't mean food manufacturers aren't putting this stuff into the processed foods you buy. Always read the labels!

Avoid: hydrogenated oil, partially hydrogenated oil, margarine, vegetable shortening and fried foods.

"Red Light Fat": Standard Vegetable Oils

For reasons we explained in chapter 1, these highly refined oils are not healthy and should not be used. Don't buy processed products that contain these oils.

- Corn oil
- Cottonseed oil
- Peanut oil
- "Pure" vegetable oil
- Safflower oil (high-oleic safflower oil is acceptable)
- Sesame seed oil
- Soybean oil
- Sunflower oil (high-oleic sunflower oil is acceptable)

The Simple Oil Swap Solution

Here are some tips for eliminating highly refined vegetable oil from your diet.

1) In *no-heat* recipes use flaxseed oil, extra-virgin olive oil, expeller-pressed canola oil or expeller-pressed walnut oil in place of less healthful processed vegetable oils. In prepared convenience foods that you will not be heating, look for expeller-pressed canola oil, expeller-pressed walnut oil or extra-virgin olive oil in the listing of ingredients. Avoid convenience foods that have been made using standard vegetable oils and trans fats.
2) For recipes *requiring heat* use extra-virgin olive oil, butter, extra-virgin coconut oil, or the high-oleic versions of canola oil, sunflower oil and safflower oil instead of standard vegetable oils. In prepared convenience foods that have been heated or that you will be heating, look for these more healthful oils and fats in the listing of ingredients instead of standard vegetable oils and trans fats.

BOTTOM LINE ————————————————————————

Use healthful alternatives to standard processed vegetable oils.

The "Yellow Light" Fat: Saturated Fat

We call saturated fat a "Yellow Light" fat because, although saturated fats found in butter, red meat and cheese can be hazardous to your health, these fats may be included in moderation as part of the Gold Coast Cure. The key word here is "moderation." A little bit of saturated fat will have no meaningful effect on your health, a little bit more will harm your health, and a lot more can be downright deadly. A good rule of thumb is to make sure all the foods you eat that contain saturated fat are nutrient-rich, all-natural whole foods. In other words, try to make every food containing saturated fat count nutritionally. Because saturated fat can add up fast, you need to keep track of your daily total saturated fat intake. This is the *only* counting you have to do while following the Cure.

The saturated fats you eat should come from nutrient-dense animal foods, occasional all-natural "sweet treats" and natural vegetable sources. *Healthy people should eat no more than 20 grams of saturated fat each day. People who already have a health condition related to their blood vessels, such as heart disease, and people who have any condition related to inflammation such as asthma, osteoarthritis, allergies or multiple sclerosis must aim to eat no more than 15 grams of saturated fat per day.*

You don't need to count the saturated fat found in non-animal foods like nuts and all-natural nut butters, seeds and seed butters, olives, avocado and extra-virgin olive oil. You also don't have to count the saturated fat in the healthful oils we list in chapter 5 because these oils contain good fat. You also don't have to count the saturated fat found in fish or shellfish.

A Simple Trick to Limit Your Saturated Fat

We find it's easiest to stick to our saturated fat gram budget when we avoid snacking on foods that contain saturated fat and we avoid saturated fat completely during one of the three main meals we eat each day. For example, if we include saturated fat as part of our breakfast (eggs, perhaps) and dinner (filet mignon or cheese) we avoid eating any other food containing saturated fat either for lunch or as a snack. This way we only have to add up our saturated fat grams twice a day. You can use whatever trick works best for you, but you must stick to the saturated fat gram budget we prescribe if you want to enjoy optimal health.

While there are many dietary sources of saturated fat, there are only three foods that contain enough saturated fat to justify worrying about. These are the *only* three types of saturated fat you have to count on the Cure:

Animal Products Other Than Fish and Shellfish

Saturated fat is found naturally in animal products, including meats, chicken, turkey, eggs, milks, cheeses and butter. Dark meat chicken and turkey contain more saturated fat than white meat. Because fatty cuts of meat contain more saturated fat than leaner cuts, always choose lean cuts of beef, lamb, pork, veal and game whenever you shop for red meat. Because meat contains nutrients that are not readily available in most vegetable products, there is no need to eliminate red meats from your diet so long as you count their saturated fat content toward your daily budget.

Processed and Prepared Food

You'll find saturated fat in many processed foods. Luckily, government health organizations require food processing firms to include the saturated fat content on the labeling of all their processed, packaged foods. Read these labels. Saturated fat content is listed on the label directly underneath the total fat content. Monitor your portion size of these foods. Every bite counts toward your daily saturated fat limit.

Tropical Vegetable Oils

Some vegetable products naturally contain large amounts of saturated fat. Vegetable oil sources of saturated fat include coconut oil, cocoa butter, palm oil and palm kernel oil. Research is ongoing as to whether vegetable sources of saturated fat are as harmful as animal sources of saturated fat. Our suspicion is the vegetable sources are less harmful only because the vegetarian sources, as long as they are not processed, contain more nutrients. Vegetable sources of saturated fat contain some of the same healthful vitamins, minerals, antioxidants and phytochemicals as are found in the nutrient-rich healthy carbohydrate foods we discuss in chapter 4.

However, until more research is available we recommend eating all tropical sources of saturated fat sparingly. This should not be too difficult because there are many tasty, more healthful alternatives to those few vegetable oils that are high in saturated fat.

Cure-Approved Saturated Fat Foods

All of the following foods contain nutrients in addition to saturated fat so all of them may be included in moderation as part of the Gold Coast Cure. Just remember to stick to your saturated fat budget of 20 grams a day for healthy people, 15 grams a day if you have a heart condition or an inflammatory condition. You must count the saturated fat in all of the following foods:

Butter

One tablespoon of butter contains 7 grams of saturated fat.

Admittedly, butter does make food taste better. Luckily butter isn't as bad for you as you may think. It's far more healthful than standard margarine, and it contains important micronutrients and antioxidants such as vitamin A, vitamin E and selenium.

A little bit of butter goes a long way. One teaspoon of butter contains only 2½ grams of saturated fat, yet this teaspoon is generally sufficient to add great flavor to an entire serving of vegetables or an entire side dish of whole grains. Ideally, butter should be used only for cooking and baking. If you use butter frequently as a spread on whole grain breads and rolls, it's best to find an acceptable low-saturated-fat alternative. Peanut butter, extra-virgin olive oil and tahini are good choices. If you're really after the butter flavor, try whipped butter instead. Whipped butter contains significantly less saturated fat than regular butter given an identical volume of product. Whipped butter tastes just like regular butter, but the texture is fluffier and lighter.

Two heart-healthy alternatives to butter are Smart Balance and Earth Balance, which we mentioned earlier in this chapter. While butter contains 2½ grams of saturated fat per teaspoon, these heart-healthy alternatives contain only 2½ grams of saturated fat per tablespoon. They taste delicious, and they really do improve your cholesterol profile as claimed on the packaging. Both of these products are far better for your health than either butter or standard margarine.

Spreads fortified with plant stanols and plant sterols have also been shown to reduce cholesterol levels and improve your cholesterol profile.[3] If you purchase these products make sure they don't contain any partially hydrogenated oil or hydrogenated oil in their list of ingredients. The same company that makes Smart Balance recently introduced Smart Balance Omega Plus spread, which contains plant sterols and essential omega-3 fat (discussed in more detail in chapter 5) with no trans fat.

Low-Fat (1% or 2%) Milk, Low-Fat Yogurt and Keifir

One cup of 2% milk or low-fat yogurt contains roughly 3 grams of saturated fat.

With the exception of the occasional gourmet cheese and butter, we do not recommend full-fat dairy products because the high amounts of saturated fat they contain tend to cancel out their potential health benefits. This having been said, a little bit of fat does dramatically improve the taste and usefulness of most dairy products. You do not need to use fat-free dairy products unless you truly prefer their taste or consistency.

Low-fat (1% or 2%) milk, low-fat yogurt and kefir, a great-tasting product available at the natural foods stores, are all wonderful sources of protein. These foods are also some of the richest dietary sources of calcium available. One cup of milk provides at least 30 percent of your daily calcium requirement. Try to get accustomed to 1% milk, which is better for your health than 2% milk. One percent milk contains only 1½ grams of saturated fat per cup as compared with the 3 grams of saturated fat found in 1 cup of 2% milk.

Finally, be careful when you buy yogurt. Many commercially available brands contain lots of added empty-calorie carbohydrates such as sugar syrups, fruit juice concentrates and corn syrup. Many fat-free flavored yogurts are very high in sugar. It's far better to buy plain, low-fat yogurt and sweeten it yourself with fresh fruit, frozen fruit or a bit of Splenda. As a quick rule of thumb, if the low-fat yogurt brand you select contains more than about 130 calories per 8-ounce serving, you should assume it contains too much added sugar.

Do You Get Enough Calcium?

Most of us don't consume anywhere near the amount of calcium we need for optimum health. This is especially true for women. Calcium is crucial for building and maintaining bone mass and preventing osteoporosis.

Research from the Nutrition Institute at the University of Tennessee, Knoxville, shows calcium-rich diets help your body burn more fat when compared with calcium-poor diets.[4] These researchers theorize that calcium may suppress the production of calcitriol, a hormone that encourages fat cells to store fat while at the same time suppressing fat burning.

If you're lactose intolerant yet still want to enjoy dairy products, try lactose-free milk, yogurt and kefir. These foods contain live bacteria that help digest lactose. The "friendly" bacteria *Lactobacillus acidophilus* found in yogurt and kefir allow your gut to develop a more healthful bacterial balance. These friendly bacteria take up space and use up food sources that would otherwise be used to support the growth of harmful bacteria that are capable of causing infections. The *Lactobacillus acidophilus* bacteria in yogurt are especially helpful for preserving natural bacterial balance in your body during and shortly after a course of antibiotics. If you're prone to yeast infections and urinary tract infections, consider eating yogurt or kefir on a daily basis.

Even if you are totally intolerant of all dairy products, there are plenty of other whole foods sources of calcium you can enjoy while on the Cure:

Food	Calcium Content
1 ounce almonds	80 mg
1 cup black beans	47 mg
½ cup broccoli	35 mg
½ cup kale	47 mg
1 cup navy beans	128 mg
3 ounces sardines *(with bones)*	92 mg
1 ounce sunflower seeds	34 mg
½ cup sweet potatoes	35 mg
½ cup tofu	130 mg

Cheese

One quarter cup of shredded full-fat cheese contains roughly 5 grams of saturated fat.

One quarter cup of low-fat cheese contains roughly 3 grams of saturated fat.

Who doesn't love cheese? When enjoyed in moderation, cheese is most definitely part of the Gold Coast Cure. Cheese is relatively rich in protein and a very good source of calcium. Low-fat products contain about half the saturated fat while sacrificing very little in taste, so look for "low-fat" or "part-skim" cheeses and save full-fat cheeses for the occasional splurge. We recommend that you avoid "fat-free" cheeses. Besides tasting like damp cardboard, fat-free, highly artificial cheese-like foods typically contain very little actual cheese, very few nutrients and many unhealthy ingredients.

Pork, Veal, Lamb, Game, Beef, Dark Meat Turkey and Dark Meat Chicken

A 4-ounce, palm-size serving of "extra lean" versions of these meats contains about 4 grams of saturated fat.

By now we all know how important it is to reduce our consumption of red meat. But, again, reduce does not mean eliminate. Instead we recommend you eat moderately sized portions of lean cuts of meats once or twice a week as part of a well-balanced diet.

Purchase only the leanest cuts of beef (tenderloin, filet and sirloin), then meticulously trim off all visible fat. Completely avoid standard sausages and standard bacon strips because they contain too much saturated fat and too few nutrients to justify eating. Turkey sausage and Canadian bacon, unlike regular bacon, are reasonably low in saturated fat and may be eaten occasionally as part of a healthy diet as long as you count the saturated fat content toward your daily allowance.

Dark meat turkey and chicken are both allowed on the Cure, but be aware that dark meat contains more than twice as much saturated fat as white meat. Also, much of the saturated fat in chicken and turkey is found right under the skin. We suggest you only eat skinless, white meat chicken and turkey.

If you want to obtain absolute optimal health and you have the time and money, we encourage you to buy grass-fed as opposed to grain-fed poultry and meats. Organic, grass-fed animals are leaner, contain two to three times more omega-3 fat than meat from grain-fed animals, and are free of antibiotics and growth hormones. For more information on the health benefits of eating grass-fed meat as well as suggestions on where to purchase this type of meat, please visit *www.eatwild.com* or *www.americangrassfedbeef.com*.

Ostrich

Beef lovers should also try ostrich. We were pleasantly surprised at how delicious and beef-like ostrich tastes. Not only is it juicy with a delicate beef flavor, it is incredibly lean and low in saturated fat. Some freeze-dried brands contain less than 2 grams of saturated fat per serving.

Skinless White Meat Chicken and Turkey

A 4-ounce, palm-size serving contains about 1½ grams of saturated fat.

As long as you don't eat the skin and you eat only the white meat, chicken and turkey are low in saturated fat. Although chicken and turkey are certainly healthy, don't go overboard. Many health-conscious people eat an excessive amount of chicken and turkey at the expense of other nutrient-rich protein foods, such as fish, soy, eggs and dairy. Don't fill up so much on chicken and turkey that you avoid eating the many other healthful foods we discuss throughout the rest of this book, especially in chapter 6.

Eggs

The average egg contains 70 calories and only 1½ grams of saturated fat.

Eggs are a nutrient-rich whole food containing protein, vitamins, minerals and lecithin. Unfortunately, because eggs are high in cholesterol, they have received an undeserved bad rap. People have believed for years that eating eggs and other cholesterol-rich foods such as shrimp significantly increases the amount of cholesterol in their bloodstream and puts them at increased risk of developing heart disease. This is just not true![5]

Eating eggs doesn't put you at increased risk of heart disease. Researchers who analyzed 912 subjects participating in the Framingham Study over a number of years found there was no significant relationship between egg consumption, blood cholesterol levels and coronary heart disease.[6] Eggs are low in saturated fat and rich in a micronutrient called lecithin that helps your body metabolize cholesterol. Eggs contain a wide variety of nutrients, including vitamins A, B_6, B_{12} and E. The egg yolk contains vitamin K, folate, iron, choline and lutein, a potent antioxidant that may help ward off age-related macular degeneration, a common cause of blindness.[7] There is no reason to avoid eating eggs.

Foods that Increase Your Cholesterol Level

Most people are unaware it is *not* the cholesterol they eat in their food that is the main culprit when it comes to the amount of cholesterol in their bloodstream. High cholesterol is mostly brought on by eating either too much saturated fat or trans fats or eating too many overly processed, empty carbohydrates. Your liver makes cholesterol from the saturated fats and trans fats you eat. And, because empty carbohydrates can be converted by your body into saturated fat, cholesterol can also be indirectly produced from any excess intake of empty carbohydrates. Excess empty-carbohydrate consumption also stimulates your body to produce large amounts of insulin, and insulin activates the main enzyme responsible for making cholesterol in your liver.

The bottom line is the actual cholesterol you eat has a minimal effect on your blood cholesterol level.

Omega-Rich Eggs

When possible, take advantage of eggs from chickens that have been fed special diets that cause them to lay eggs that are richer in the good essential omega-3 fats you will learn more about in chapter 5. One of our favorite brands of "omega-3 eggs" can be bought at almost any supermarket. Eggland's Best eggs contain 25 percent less saturated fat than regular eggs while containing three times more omega-3 fat than regular eggs. The Eggland's Best hen feed contains no animal fat, no animal byproducts, and no recycled or processed food. Eggland's Best never uses hormones or antibiotics of any kind. These eggs taste exactly the same, if not better, than regular eggs. And, if that's not enough to convince you, omega-3 enriched eggs have a favorable effect on your cholesterol profile by increasing your good HDL cholesterol level and decreasing your triglyceride level.[8]

Now that you know a little bit about the few unhealthy foods to avoid, it's time to learn about the many foods you can enjoy on the Cure lifestyle.

Part Two

Eating for Weight Loss and Health: The Foods That Slim and Heal

Saying Yes to Healthy Carbs

The vast majority of carbohydrates are perfectly healthful and strongly encouraged on the Cure. In fact, there are far more good carbs to choose from than there are empty carbs to avoid. But in order to lose weight and be healthy, you need to eat *nutrient-rich* carbs.

The Produce Section

All fruits and *all* vegetables are allowed on the Gold Coast Cure. The antioxidants and phytochemicals found in fruits and vegetables protect you from heart disease, stroke, cancer, cataracts, eye disease and a host of diseases affecting almost any organ that relies on blood flow to survive. The bad LDL cholesterol everyone worries so much about does most of its damage after it is oxidized; the more antioxidants you eat, the less damage cholesterol can do to your blood vessels (this applies no matter how high or how low your cholesterol level may be). Fruits and vegetables are an extremely important component of any diet because they are nature's richest food sources of antioxidants.

Fruits

Fruit is Mother Nature's ultimate nutrient-packed fast food: Simply wash and eat. We realize some diet gurus are against fruit; that's absolutely ridiculous. Fruits are one of the very best sources of lasting energy. They're packed with nutrients, phytochemicals, antioxidants and folate and are rich in fiber. Try to eat a wide variety of fruits of all different colors to maximize your exposure to the broadest range of vitamins, minerals, antioxidants and micronutrients.

BOTTOM LINE ────────────────────────────────────

All whole fruits are good.

Fresh Fruit Versus Frozen, Canned and Dried

FROZEN: Fresh fruit usually tastes best, but frozen fruit is every bit as nutritious.

DRIED: Dried fruits are also acceptable, but be sure to read the label to make sure there is no added sugar or oils. If you're very active, consider increasing your consumption of dried fruit to increase your carbohydrate intake. Athletes who eat dried fruit enjoy increased energy without feeling bloated or weighed down.

CANNED: We advise *against* eating canned fruits because they are almost always packed in refined, sugary syrups. Be sure to scan the list of ingredients when purchasing canned or packaged fruit. The ingredient list must include only 100 percent fruit without added sugar. Avoid canned fruit unless the only ingredients are fruit, water and perhaps a preservative or two.

BOTTOM LINE ────────────────────────────────────

Eat more fresh, frozen and dried fruit. Avoid canned fruit.

Vegetables

We are horrified that many low-carb diet gurus classify some vegetables, such as carrots, as "bad carbs." Ridiculous. Vegetables—carrots included—are loaded with fiber, vitamins, minerals, antioxidants and disease-fighting phytochemicals. If you want to achieve optimum health, you must eat a wide variety of vegetables frequently. Trust us, you won't get fat eating carrots. *All* vegetables are healthful carbohydrates that offer tremendous nutritional and antioxidant bang for a minimal calorie buck.

You should eat at least one large serving of vegetables at lunch and at dinner. One serving is about 1 cup (or the size of your closed fist). While fresh vegetables usually taste best, using frozen vegetables is a great time-saver. Interestingly, frozen vegetables actually retain more nutrients than all but the very freshest "fresh" vegetables. Because modern commercial growers have such sophisticated packaging methods, there is hardly any time for nutrients to be lost prior to freezing and packaging vegetables for shipment to the grocery store. Canned vegetables are perfectly fine, too.

BOTTOM LINE ———————————————————————
All vegetables are good, whether fresh, frozen or canned. Eat a 1-cup serving at lunch and dinner.

Three Vegetable Superstars

While all vegetables are healthy, the following ones provide such extensive health benefits that we believe you cannot attain truly optimal health without *intentionally* including them in your diet.

Power Veggie #1: Garlic The pyramid builders in ancient Egypt ate garlic daily for strength, endurance and general health. Garlic has been proven to aid in the prevention of heart disease. Garlic contains a compound called methyl allyl trisulfide that lowers blood pressure by dilating blood vessel walls and can also significantly reduce your blood cholesterol level.[1] Garlic lowers your bad LDL cholesterol level and prevents the LDL cholesterol in your blood from oxidizing. Oxidized LDL cholesterol is bad news because it encourages plaque deposits on your arterial lining, which leads to heart disease. Because of its effect on your blood cholesterol level, garlic helps prevent most types of stroke, all types of vascular senility, heart attacks, kidney disease and claudication. In Germany, garlic supplements are actually registered and prescribed as drugs for use against arteriosclerosis.

BOTTOM LINE ─────────────────────────────
Eat garlic at least three or four times a week.

Power Veggie #2: Tomatoes Tomatoes are rich in nutrients such as the antioxidant vitamins C and E, potassium, folic acid, beta carotene, and lycopene. Although lycopene is most popular for its ability to reduce prostate cancer, this powerful antioxidant has also been shown to reduce cancer rates in the cervix, mouth, pharynx, esophagus, stomach, colon and rectum. Additionally, lycopene is one phytochemical thought to be *independently* protective against heart attacks.[2]

Cooking and canning tomatoes does not destroy lycopene so there's no need to eat raw tomatoes if you don't like them. Tomato sauce is fine, too. Because lycopene is fat soluble, you need to eat tomato foods in combination with some type of dietary fat, such as olive oil, nuts or butter, in order to enjoy maximal benefit.

BOTTOM LINE ─────────────────────────────
Eat at least one serving of tomato every week.

Power Veggie #3: Broccoli Broccoli is rich in antioxidants and has been shown to be effective in fighting lung, colon and breast cancer. Recent studies have also linked eating broccoli to a reduced risk of cervical cancer. The phytochemical indole-3 carbinol found in broccoli assists with the conversion of certain "bad" estrogens in your blood into more benign "good" estrogens. This shift in estrogen metabolism is measurable and significant,[3] providing protection against hormone-responsive cancers such as breast cancer and colon cancer.

One cup of broccoli supplies a hefty dose of calcium and contains more vitamin C than an orange. Broccoli is also rich in vitamin K, a substance necessary for maintaining healthy bones.

BOTTOM LINE

Eat broccoli at least once a week.

Gold Coast–Approved Dense Carbohydrates

Aside from fruits and vegetable, dense carbohydrates are integral to a healthy diet. The "dense carbohydrates" category of foods consists of whole grains, beans, legumes and starchy vegetables such as yams and potatoes.

Whole Grains

What makes whole grains so good for you? Whole grains contain fiber; vitamin E and the B vitamins; minerals such as magnesium, selenium, copper, manganese and zinc; and disease-fighting phyto-chemicals—nutrients your body needs. Remember, nutrient-rich foods fill you up, not out.

Unfortunately, many people think whole grains are bland and boring and difficult to make (not so as you'll see in chapter 16). Try them and you'll see: there are a wide variety of whole grains that are filling, slimming and taste great, too.

You can find whole grains at your local supermarket, although you may wish to go to the natural foods store to find a wider variety. Most supermarkets carry brown rice, wild rice, barley, whole-grain pasta, whole-grain bread, old-fashioned oats and a few other whole-grain cereals. The other whole grains on our list can be readily obtained at a natural foods store, and almost all may be bought inexpensively in bulk. In our "Kitchen Shape-Up" in chapter 8, we give you an overview of what to buy at the natural foods store.

Almost all whole grains are low-priced, simple to prepare and delicious to eat. It's best to vary the grains you eat as much as possible. By doing so you won't get bored and you'll obtain the widest possible range of nutrients. People with gluten intolerance or wheat allergies can follow the Cure by rotating gluten-free and wheat-free grains and flours. In alphabetical order, here is a listing of some of the healthy, versatile whole grains we use regularly in our cooking:

Amaranth: A mildly spicy, South American whole grain with a slightly peppery flavor, amaranth is rich in calcium, protein and iron, and can be served either as a side dish or as a cereal. It develops a creamy texture when cooked and makes a great high-fiber soup thickener.

Barley: Relatively easy to find and gluten-free, whole barley can be used to make tasty pilafs, soups, stews and cold vegetable salads. Because of its neutral flavor, fiber-rich barley can be used instead of white rice in many of your favorite recipes. Seek out nutritious whole-grain "brown" barley; avoid processed "polished" barley if possible.

Brown Rice: This grain is gluten-free and nutrient rich. Choose either long- or short-grain brown rice but *avoid* the refined white stuff entirely. If you have never tried brown rice, you will be pleasantly surprised by its rich, nutty flavor. Add interest to your meal by combining brown rice with wild rice, chopped nuts, dried cranberries, finely chopped vegetables, your favorite fresh or dried herbs, butter or extra-virgin olive oil, and a bit of salt and pepper.

Bulgar: Sold precooked and ready to use, this traditional Middle

Eastern whole grain is used to create dishes such as tabbouleh and kibbeh. Purchase fine or medium-ground bulgar for tabbouleh. Use more coarsely ground bulgar for making pilafs.

Buckwheat: Buckwheat is gluten-free and has a nutty flavor. Whole buckwheat flour makes wonderfully healthful pancakes and waffles. Roasted buckwheat is also called "kasha."

Corn and Stone-Ground Cornmeal: Stone-ground cornmeal is excellent in cornbread, polenta and tortillas, but you need to avoid processed, nutrient-poor, fiber-poor "de-germed" cornmeal. Always read the product label and make sure there are at least 2 grams of fiber per 25 grams of carbohydrate in any packaged corn product you purchase.

Couscous: Purchase only whole-wheat couscous, otherwise you'll miss out on most of the fiber and the nutrients. Look for the word "whole" on the box.

Kamut: A high-protein variety of wheat berry, kamut has an appealing chewy texture when cooked and can be made into a variety of side dishes.

Millet: Rich in B vitamins, copper and iron, this gluten-free whole grain makes a great side dish. You can serve it as a breakfast cereal with a little milk or soy milk, plus fresh fruit and chopped nuts. Because of its mild, pasta-like taste, kids love it.

Oats: Oatmeal's health benefits have been published in major medical journals. Oat fiber has been specifically shown to possess heart-healthy benefits, including a reduced bad LDL cholesterol level in your bloodstream.[4] Whole grain oats contain the antioxidant vitamin E, seven B vitamins, and nine minerals including calcium and iron. When shopping for oatmeal, avoid "instant" refined versions and opt for the unrefined "old-fashioned" oats.

Quinoa: Quinoa is the queen of grains when it comes to protein, iron and calcium. This gluten-free grain has a mild taste and can be used as a side dish to meat, fish or poultry; stuffed in bell peppers or tomatoes; used in puddings and stir-fries; or tossed into soups or salads. As a simple, quick side dish, top cooked quinoa with either extra-virgin olive oil or flaxseed oil and freshly grated Parmesan cheese.

Whole Wheat: With so many types of wheat for sale, it's easy to get confused. All of the following wheat products are nutrient rich and may be eaten with confidence.

- **Whole-wheat flour** should *always* be used instead of enriched, refined "white" flour and is excellent for making muffins, cakes and breads. (If you're allergic to wheat, look for alternative nutritious whole-grain flours such as amaranth flour, whole-barley flour, whole-oat flour and triticale flour. These flours can be purchased at the natural foods store.)

- **Wheat bran** is an outstanding source of fiber. It's readily available at most grocery stores and may be added to baked goods and cereals to increase the overall fiber content. One quarter cup of wheat bran contains a whopping 8 grams of fiber!

- **Wheat berries** are chewy in texture and can be added to salads or rice pilaf. (See the recipe section.)

- **Cracked wheat** is similar in texture to wheat berries. We like cracked wheat as a cereal in the morning with a little soy milk or low-fat milk, fresh fruit and chopped nuts.

- **Wheat germ** is loaded with vitamin E, folic acid, various B vitamins, fiber and essential fat. You can add it to muffins, breakfast cereals, breads, meatloaf, meatballs and cookies. Sprinkle it on top of yogurt and fruit, or on top of your favorite all-natural ice cream. Young kids especially like the crispy texture of wheat germ and will not suspect it's "health" food unless you tell them.

Cooking Whole Grains

If you're new to whole grains, we recommend you buy an inexpensive rice cooker with a timer. The rice cooker will cook your whole grains perfectly, eliminating the need for you to watch the pot.

If you have no room for another gadget in your kitchen, simply boil water, add the whole grain, then wait until the kernels are tender. Prep time varies depending on the grain. (Chapter 16 includes a quick reference guide for cooking many of the most popular whole grains.)

You can cook whole grains ahead of time then slightly salt, cover and refrigerate them for up to three days. By adding distinctive cheeses, oils, spices and fresh herbs at the last minute, you can make a new dish every night. Simply reheat the dish in the microwave immediately prior to serving, or lightly sauté the cooked grain in a skillet with a little extra-virgin olive oil.

BOTTOM LINE ————————————————————————————

Learn to cook whole grains. Serve them instead of overprocessed white-flour carbs.

Pass the Whole-Grain Bread, Please

We encourage you to enjoy bread but be sure you're always eating "whole" grain bread that contains no trans fats. The first item on the ingredient list of any bread label must either be a whole grain or some type of whole-grain flour. The bread should contain absolutely no hydrogenated or partially hydrogenated oils.

We are huge fans of the Alvarado Street Bakery, which makes wonderful breads. One of our favorites is called California-Style Complete Protein Bread. Food manufacturers must list the ingredients contained in their products in descending order according to quantity. Notice how many whole grains are included in the list of ingredients that follows and notice how the very first ingredient is a whole grain:

An Example of Good Bread:

ALVARADO STREET BAKERY
CALIFORNIA-STYLE COMPLETE PROTEIN BREAD

INGREDIENTS: ORGANICALLY GROWN HIGH PROTEIN SPROUTED WHEAT BERRIES, FILTERED WATER, MILLET, CORN, ROLLED OATS, SOYBEANS, LENTILS, BARLEY, MALT, PURE HONEY, GLUTEN, SEA SALT, FRESH YEAST, SOY-BASED LECITHIN

Being able to identify "bad bread" is just as important. Without naming names, we can tell you one particular bad bread is a best-selling brand being advertised inappropriately as a health food product. Just the first two ingredients—unbleached, enriched wheat flour and malted barley flour—show that this bread does not even come close to being healthy. High fructose corn syrup is another "red flag" ingredient listed on the label. Again, always read the labels.

The bread we are referring to provides an excellent example of how you simply cannot rely on package advertising. This bad bread states boldly on its packaging that there are no preservatives, no artificial colors and no artificial flavors. Furthermore, the manufacturer claims the product is "cholesterol-free." While all of this may be true, if you eat this empty-calorie junk food on a regular basis, you increase your risk of obesity, heart disease, diabetes, colon cancer and a host of other health problems. On the plus side, you will, of course, not be consuming any artificial colors. Big deal!

BOTTOM LINE ————————————————————————————————
Purchase breads made with whole grains and whole-grain flours only and no trans fats.

Pleasing Pasta Lovers

Pasta is one of those foods just about everyone loves. Nevertheless, many health- and weight-conscious people avoid pasta entirely for fear it's fattening. In truth, pasta is similar to bread in that certain types of pasta are very healthy and can actually help you slim down while certain varieties are not healthy and will certainly not help you in your battle with the bulge.

It's very easy to differentiate between healthy pasta and unhealthy refined pasta by using the same skills you would use to find good bread. *Healthy pastas are made from whole grains and whole-grain flour and contain at least 2 to 3 grams of fiber per 25 grams of carbohydrate.*

Unfortunately it can be difficult to find good pasta because typical supermarket and restaurant pasta varieties are *not* healthful. Almost all standard pasta is made from refined, enriched flour or refined semolina. If you do not see the word "whole" as part of the first ingredient in the list of ingredients on the side of the box, you must assume the product is an empty-calorie pasta. While many supermarkets carry whole-wheat pasta or "blended" pasta (partially whole grain, partially refined flour), you may still have to go to the natural foods store to find a wider selection.

BOTTOM LINE ———————————————————————————

Whole-grain pasta is healthy if it contains at the very least 2 grams of fiber per 25 grams of carbohydrate.

One Potato, Two Potato

We cringe when we hear people say potatoes are "fattening" or bad for you. Potatoes, when eaten with their skins, are natural whole foods containing fiber and important nutrients such as vitamin C, iron, various B vitamins and potassium, in addition to many other healthful micronutrients and phytochemicals. A baked potato that is roughly the size of your fist contains about 35 grams of carbohdyrate and 3 grams of fiber.

Unfortunately, many people turn potatoes into unhealthy foods by removing the fiber-rich skins and then processing them into oblivion. Restaurant-style French fries are the perfect example. Instant "mashed" potatoes that have been skinned, dehydrated, reconstituted and stripped of their nutrients are another example. Finally, potatoes drowned in an excessive amount of unhealthful saturated fats such as butter, full-fat sour cream, full-fat cheese and gravy will not help you stay slim or healthy.

Potatoes make a great side dish when dressed with extra-virgin olive oil or flaxseed oil, herbs, spices, salsa, heart-healthy guacamole, Parmesan cheese or low-fat sour cream. If you can't imagine eating potatoes without butter, go ahead, but go easy. Another option is to top your potato with a heart-healthy spread such as Smart Balance or Earth Balance—both are low in saturated fat and free from the trans fats that make standard margarines so unhealthful.

Sweet potatoes are also good for you and should always be eaten whole, with the skin.

BOTTOM LINE ───────────────────────────────────

Whole potatoes and sweet potatoes are good for you.

Bean Cuisine

Many nutritionists feel beans are second only to whole grains in their importance as a healthful, high-energy nutrient source. Beans are filling and satisfying, and they are loaded with vitamins, minerals, phytochemicals, protein and fiber.

Their high protein content gives them an edge over other carbohydrates and makes them a staple food for vegetarians. Beans also help lower your cholesterol levels and reduce your homocysteine level, further reducing your risk of heart disease. The amino acids glutamine and arginine found in beans help reduce your blood pressure and help your intestines protect you against illnesses caused by bacterial overgrowth.

A Significant Protein Source for Vegans

Because beans are so rich in protein, vegans eat them in combination with certain other foods in order to create complete protein meals that are just as nourishing as the chicken and steak meals you might be more familiar with. While beans alone do not fulfill your body's requirements for protein, the protein you get from eating beans in *combination* with any of the following foods is just as complete and just as good for you as the protein you would get if you chose to eat milk, red meat, eggs or chicken:

- Brown rice
- Corn
- Nuts
- Seeds
- Wheat

While we do not recommend a vegan diet for everyone, it is entirely possible to be 100 percent healthy on a vegan diet.

Beans, like whole grains, may be prepared in bulk well ahead of time. In chapter 16, we include a quick reference for cooking beans and several quick, easy, tasty bean-based recipes.

To get around the convenience quandary, keep a bowl of cooked beans in the fridge so you can add them to any meal in a flash. Cooked beans last approximately three to four days if they are covered, lightly salted and refrigerated. Also, there is absolutely nothing wrong with buying canned beans. If you use canned beans, do what chefs do and wash them thoroughly with water in a strainer before preparing them in order to eliminate any trace of "canned" flavor. Beans are exceptionally versatile and should be added liberally to soups, salads, side dishes and grain pilafs. And don't forget about other "legume" foods such as peas and lentils.

BOTTOM LINE ————————————————————————

Beans are always good.

Gold Coast–Approved
Packaged Carbohydrate Foods

You can eat packaged crackers, cold cereals and snack foods as long as they are made from whole grains and as long as they don't contain processed vegetable oils (such as corn oil and "pure" vegetable oil) and trans fats (such as vegetable shortening and hydrogenated or partially hydrogenated oils). Enriched flour is *not* allowed. *Packaged carbohydrate foods should always contain at least 2 grams, and ideally 3 grams, of fiber per 25 grams of carbohydrate.* The carbohydrate content per serving and the fiber content per serving are required by law to appear on the package labeling.

BOTTOM LINE ———————————————————————————

Packaged "carb" products must contain at least 2 grams, and ideally 3 grams, of fiber per 25 grams of carbohydrates. Read the labels.

Concluding Carbohydrates

By now you should have a complete understanding of the difference between healthy, nutrient-rich carbs and empty carbs. You should also be able to breeze through your local grocery store, pick any carbohydrate product up off the shelf and know whether it's a good or bad carb.

In the next chapter, we'll introduce you to the healing and slimming fats.

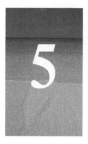

Saying Yes to Healthy Fats: Essential and Monounsaturated Fats

We've given you the lowdown on the bad fats. Now it's time for the good news. There are many Green Light fats that have the power to reduce inflammation in your body and improve a broad range of health conditions while helping you slim down.

"Green Light" Fat #1: Omega-3 Essential Fats

The omega-3 fats are the most powerful anti-inflammatory substances available without a prescription. Omega-3 fats are used by your body *only* to make good anti-inflammatory substances called prostaglandins. Increasing your consumption of omega-3 fats helps prevent, stabilize and even reverse a huge range of inflammation-mediated conditions such as asthma, arthritis, multiple sclerosis, heart disease, vascular dementia, psoriasis and allergies.

Food Sources of Healthful Omega-3 Essential Fat

Truly Rich Sources of Omega-3 Fat

- Fatty fish
- Fish oil supplements
- Flaxseeds
- Flax oil

Foods Containing Moderate Amounts of Healthful Omega-3 Fat

- Non-fatty fish
- Shellfish
- Canola oil (expeller-pressed, unheated canola oil only)
- Walnuts
- Expeller-pressed walnut oil that has not been heated
- Unrefined whole soy products such as tofu and whole soybeans

NOTE: *Soybean oil does not contain omega-3 fat in a useful form.*

Go Fish!

Fish is a fantastic nutrient-dense food that's rich in complete protein and low in saturated fat. Fish offers an assortment of vitamins and minerals, including antioxidant vitamin E, most of the B vitamins, copper, iodine, phosphorous, selenium and zinc.

However, the main benefit you get from fish is the preformed DHA and EPA contained within its flesh. EPA and DHA are the two omega-3 fats that are the most useful for fighting inflammation. Fatty fish and the fish oils gleaned from fatty fish represent the only commercially available significant food sources of EPA and DHA.

While it's possible for your body to make EPA and DHA from another omega-3 fat called LNA found in flaxseeds and flax oil, it's impossible for your body to make enough EPA and DHA no matter how much LNA you eat. For this reason, you need to eat fish, or, at the very least, you need to take fish oil supplements even if you also eat the flaxseeds and flax oil we recommend. (Fish oil supplements are discussed in more detail in chapter 11.)

You can eat as few as two servings of fish per week as long as you supplement your diet with high-quality fish oil. We strongly encourage everyone to supplement with fish oil; in real life it's very difficult to obtain the suggested optimal intake of 3 grams per day of combined EPA and DHA eating food alone. Regardless of the source, fish or fish oil, the benefits of EPA and DHA are identical.

BOTTOM LINE ───────────────────────────────────

Fish and fish oil are the best sources of omega-3 fats.

Get Fabulously Fit with Flax

Flax is nature's richest source of LNA, a special type of omega-3 fat that is *not* found in fish. Although flax is rich in LNA, flax is not a direct source of either EPA or DHA. Because EPA, DHA and LNA are all equally important for your health, you can only obtain optimal health by eating both fish and flax.

The LNA in flax is needed for overall cardiovascular health and the prevention of inflammation-mediated conditions including asthma, multiple sclerosis, arthritis, fibromyalgia, allergies, vascular dementia, heart disease, acne and psoriasis.

The LNA found in flax can also help you trim down because your body doesn't store essential fats as body fat. Instead, your body uses essential fats to repair its millions of cell membranes, build anti-inflammatory mediators and maintain a healthy metabolism. And if you don't consume enough essential fats such as LNA, your body will not be able to burn stored fat for energy and you'll have a difficult time losing weight.

While you're whittling your waistline with LNA, you'll also be improving the condition of your skin and your overall appearance. Anti-inflammatory omega-3 fats help clear your complexion, soften your skin and strengthen your hair and nails. Many top dermatologists and avant-garde health skin-care professionals recommend dietary flax to their clients.

How Much Flax Is Enough?

It's easy to attain optimal amounts of the essential omega-3 fat LNA. All you need to do is add either 1 tablespoon of flaxseed oil or 3 tablespoons of ground flaxseeds to your daily diet.

How Do I Get My "Flax Fix"?

FLAXSEED OIL: You can purchase flax oil at any natural food store, any health food store and most vitamin shops. Because it's difficult to mass-produce flaxseed oil, most supermarkets don't stock it, and it's somewhat more costly than most oils. However, you only need 1 tablespoon of flaxseed oil a day, so one bottle can go a long way.

You must be selective when purchasing flaxseed oil. Because flaxseed oil has a limited shelf life, it's important to choose a product with a pressing date no more than four months in the past. Be sure to look for high-quality refrigerated flaxseed oil that has been expeller-pressed and fully protected from heat, light and air during the packaging process.

Strictly observe any "best before" date on the label. High-volume sellers usually stock fresh products, but it's still a good idea to check the "best before" date. Fresh flaxseed oil is nearly odorless with a light, airy, mildly nutty taste. Rancid flaxseed oil has a fishy odor and an unpleasant taste. Eating rancid flaxseed oil is worse for your health than not eating flax at all, so if you open a bottle and determine the oil isn't fresh, discard or return it. We have come to fully trust Barlean's Organic Oils as our primary source for consistently fresh, consistently delicious flaxseed oil.

Never heat flaxseed oil. The essential fat LNA is highly heat-sensitive and cannot withstand high-heat cooking temperatures.

GROUND FLAXSEEDS: Ground flaxseeds, also known as linseeds, are an alternative to flax oil. Three tablespoons of ground flaxseeds contain just about the same amount of LNA as 1 tablespoon of flax oil. Your body can't derive the full benefit of LNA if you consume flaxseeds whole, so ground (milled) flaxseed is the way to go.

You can buy ground flaxseeds at the natural foods store, or you can grind whole flaxseeds yourself with a coffee grinder. The Barlean's Organic Oils company makes a fabulous ground flaxseed product called Forti-Flax. To preserve freshness we suggest you store ground flaxseeds in your freezer unless the package has not yet been opened. Flaxseeds that have not yet been ground may be stored safely at room temperature.

Flaxseeds do have some advantages over flaxseed oil. You can heat, cook and bake with flaxseeds, and they provide a full spectrum of nutritional benefits in addition to providing the omega-3 fat LNA: protein, carbs, antioxidants and lots of fiber.

Flaxseeds are also nature's richest food source of lignans, potent antioxidants that fight free radical damage and act as phytoestrogens. Lignans and a few other naturally occurring phytoestrogens provide protection against hormone-sensitive cancers such as breast cancer,[1] ovarian cancer, uterine cancer,[2] prostate cancer[3] and even colon cancer. Flaxseeds are potent anticancer medicine.

Flax in the Kitchen

Flaxseed Oil

Adding flaxseed oil to your diet doesn't require a major lifestyle overhaul and doesn't demand any sacrifice in food flavor. It's very easy to substitute the less healthful oils you currently use for flaxseed oil in a wide array of *no-heat recipes.*

Be sure to store flaxseed oil in your refrigerator and keep it in its original opaque container. Flaxseed oil is sensitive to air and spoilage so if you make one of our flax-based vinaigrette dressings or one of our no-heat recipes using flaxseed oil, be sure to store it in a tightly sealed container in your refrigerator for no more than about two days. Finally, use your entire bottle of flaxseed oil within three to six weeks of the purchase date. These precautions are mandatory, or you will be taking your flaxseed oil for nothing.

The mild, slightly nutty flavor of flaxseed oil marries well with a wide assortment of foods. Try using flaxseed oil instead of butter to flavor vegetables, grain pilafs, rice and beans, whole grain pasta or potatoes after they've been cooked and are still warm. Short-term exposure to this low heat won't damage flax oil. Here are ten tasty options to try:

1) Use flax oil to make vinaigrettes or mix it with balsamic vinegar and splash the dressing over a salad of fresh buffalo mozzarella, tomatoes and fresh basil.
2) Use flax oil in homemade hummus.
3) Dip whole grain bread into a saucer filled with flax oil, freshly grated Parmesan cheese and coarse ground pepper.
4) Create chilled whole-grain pasta and bean salads topped with roasted red peppers, crumbled light feta cheese and flax oil.
5) Grill a low-fat cheese and roasted vegetable sandwich, then drizzle flax oil on top.
6) Drizzle flaxseed oil on top of your cooked vegetables.
7) Use flaxseed oil instead of butter on your baked potatoes.
8) Mix flaxseed oil in a cold gazpacho soup.
9) Make a southwestern-style black bean salsa using flaxseed oil, crushed garlic, fresh tomato salsa, black beans, cilantro and lime.
10) Drizzle flaxseed oil over cooked brown rice, barley or amaranth, and top with freshly shaved Parmesan cheese.

The possibilities are almost endless. Refer to our Gold Coast Cookbook section for recipe ideas.

As stated earlier, *it is imperative not to cook with flaxseed oil or any other oil rich in essential fats.* That means no baking, no sautéing and no frying with flaxseed oil. Cook instead with heat-stable, extra-virgin olive oil, butter, extra-virgin coconut oil, high-oleic canola oil, or the high-oleic versions of either sunflower oil or safflower oil.

Flaxseeds

Ground flaxseeds are great when mixed with yogurt, cottage cheese and hot cereals. You can add them to casseroles, meat loaf, meatballs, turkey burgers, whole-grain pancake or waffle batter, whole-grain breads and muffins. They're great whipped into fruit smoothies and sprinkled into cakes and cookies.

Ground flaxseeds make a delicious, healthful substitute for the cooking oil, butter, margarine and shortening called for in many baked goods recipes. Use ground flaxseeds as a substitute for cooking oil, butter, margarine or shortening at a ratio of 2 to 1. In other words use 1 cup of ground flaxseeds to replace ½ cup of butter or ½ cup margarine. If you don't want to replace the butter entirely, just replace half the butter. In other words, use ½ cup ground flaxseeds and ¼ cup butter in a recipe calling for ½ cup butter. We suggest you try some of our recipes in chapter 12 first before venturing out on your own.

Flax and Kids

Good nutrition is crucial for the proper development of your child's mind and body. Children should eat flaxseed oil or ground flaxseeds daily, too. Children who have been weaned but are under three years of age should eat about 1 teaspoon of flaxseed oil or 1 tablespoon of ground flaxseeds every day. Older children under one hundred pounds should eat 2 teaspoons of flaxseed oil a day or 2 tablespoons of ground flaxseeds daily. Children and teenagers over one hundred pounds should enjoy the standard adult serving of 1 tablespoon of flaxseed oil or 3 tablespoons of flaxseeds daily. Babies who are breast-feeding do not need to supplement with flax, though mothers undoubtedly should!

It's easy to include flax in your child's diet. Blake, our son, has no idea we sneak flaxseed oil and ground flaxseeds into one of his meals every day. For example, his whole-grain macaroni and cheese gets a drizzle of flax oil just before it is served, his whole-grain waffles are made with ground flaxseeds, and we mix ground flaxseeds in his oatmeal along with diced fruit. We even toss flaxseeds into his fruit smoothies and sprinkle them on his ice cream. Adding flax is an easy, economical way to give your child a healthy head start in life.

BOTTOM LINE ————————————————————
Eat either 1 tablespoon of flax oil or 3 tablespoons of ground flaxseeds daily.

"Green Light" Fat #2: Omega-6 Whole Foods

Unlike omega-3 essential fats, the omega-6 fats *are* found in large quantities in many commonly eaten foods. As a matter of fact, most of us already eat more omega-6 fat than we really need. The problem is we tend to get this omega-6 fat in its least healthful and heat-damaged form, as highly refined vegetable oil. Only undamaged omega-6 fats can be used by your body to make anti-inflammatory hormones and lower both your total blood cholesterol level and your bad LDL blood cholesterol level. Undamaged omega-6 fats can be beneficial to people who suffer from inflammatory conditions as long as they are not eaten in excess.

While the omega-6 fats in vegetable oil are easily damaged by heat, whole foods containing essential fat can be used for cooking because the rest of the food substance surrounds and protects the essential fat from harm. Whole foods provide the omega-6 fat you need and the nutrients you need in a 100 percent heat-safe package.

How Much Omega-6?

To get the omega-6 fat your body needs you, should eat at least one omega-6-rich whole food per day. This is not at all difficult. All of the following "whole foods" are rich in omega-6 fat:

- Sunflower seeds
- Sesame seeds
- Tahini (sesame seed butter)
- Pumpkin seeds
- Soybeans
- Dry roasted soy nuts
- Tofu
- Soy milk
- Edamame beans (soft soybeans designed for cooking)
- Wheat germ
- All natural peanut butter (must contain no hydrogenated oils)
- Dry-roasted or raw peanuts
- Walnuts
- Almonds

This list is by no means comprehensive. Almost all nuts, almost all nut butters and almost all whole grains contain at least some omega-6 fat. Nut butters are just as healthful as whole nuts as long as they don't contain added sugar, hydrogenated oil or partially hydrogenated oil. Avoid nuts and seeds that have been roasted in oil. It doesn't do you any good to buy nuts and seeds that have been cooked (roasted) in the very same vegetable oils you are specifically trying to eliminate! Dry roasted nuts and seeds are great filling and convenient snacks. If you dine out or travel frequently consider bringing a small bag along. Nuts and seeds can be discreetly tossed into any restaurant side salad.

Omega-6 Foods in the Kitchen

Omega-6 whole foods are delicious, nutritious and versatile. While it is unsafe to cook with standard vegetable oils such as corn oil, sunflower oil and soybean oil that contain omega-6 fat, you can safely cook with omega-6 whole foods. For example, you can make tofu chili, bake seeds and nuts into whole-grain breads and muffins, or use soy milk instead of milk in many recipes.

Most omega-6 whole foods are also great raw. You can sprinkle nuts and seeds into salads, cereal or yogurt. Toss sunflower seeds or edamame beans onto your salad. Sprinkle wheat germ into your cereal or use it as an ingredient in homemade whole-grain muffins. Snack on salted, roasted soybeans. Enjoy a soy-fruit smoothie. Make a Middle Eastern–style bean dip from tahini. We encourage you to experiment with new foods and new tastes!

BOTTOM LINE ――――――――――――――――――――――――――

Eat at least one omega-6 whole food every day.

"Green Light" Fat #3: Monounsaturated Fats

Monounsaturated fat is nutritious, heat-stable and heart healthy. These fats can safely provide lasting satisfaction and fullness without the dangers associated with saturated fats and trans fats. Monounsaturated fats also seem to boost your body's ability to metabolize the essential omega-3 fats. And monounsaturated fats are very versatile in the kitchen; they are heat-stable so you may cook and bake with any monounsaturated oil. Try to eat at least one serving of monounsaturated fat per day. Choose from the following sources:

Extra-Virgin Olive Oil: 1 serving = 1 tablespoon

This is by far the healthiest oil to use for cooking, hands down. Extra-virgin olive oil contains the highest percentage of heat-stable monounsaturated fat of any commercially available oil.

Avoid any olive oil that does not explicitly say "extra-virgin" or "virgin" on its container. Extra-virgin and virgin olive oils are made from the highest quality olives and are taken from the first olive pressings. A minimal amount of heat is used to obtain the first olive pressings so these extra-virgin olive oils are minimally heat-damaged even if they have been commercially processed. While a bit pricier than standard-grade "pure" olive oil, the taste, quality and health benefits are worth the price. It's perfectly fine to buy extra-virgin olive oil at the grocery store.

The antioxidants and flavonoids in extra-virgin olive oil prevent bad LDL cholesterol from oxidizing in your bloodstream. Remember, bad LDL cholesterol does most of its damage after it oxidizes. If you consume extra-virgin olive oil, you get double protection from bad cholesterol. Your LDL level goes down because of the monounsaturated fat, *and* the LDL that remains within your bloodstream is less likely to oxidize because of the antioxidants.

Olives: 1 serving = 15 small olives, 12 large olives, or ½ cup sliced olives

You get the same health benefits from eating olives whole as you do from using extra-virgin olive oil.

Expeller-Pressed Canola Oil: 1 serving = 1 tablespoon

The majority of the calories in standard canola oil comes from monounsaturated fat, but almost 30 percent of the calories come from omega-3 and omega-6 essential fat. The omega-3 and omega-6 fats are highly heat-sensitive. For this reason don't use expeller-pressed canola oil in recipes requiring heat.

Expeller-pressed canola oil is the highest quality canola oil you can buy. "Expeller-pressed" means the canola oil was not exposed to solvents during manufacturing. Unfortunately, there is no universal stamp of approval for canola oil that compares with the "extra-virgin" designation used to mark high-quality olive oil. Despite this problem, if you purchase expeller-pressed canola oil from a health foods manufacturer, you can be reasonably sure you are purchasing a high-quality product. Ideally, canola oil is a product you should purchase at the natural foods market as opposed to the local supermarket. Most standard grocery store canola oils are processed using too much heat.

Some diet books recommend incorporating canola oil into your diet as a way of obtaining more omega-3 fat. We prefer you get your omega-3 fats from flaxseeds, flaxseed oil and fish because it's far more efficient to optimize your omega ratio by eating these foods. Flaxseed oil contains almost *five* times more essential omega-3 fat than an equivalent amount of canola oil. Both oils are acceptable, but flaxseed oil is far better. Again, neither flaxseed oil nor expeller-pressed canola oil should be used for cooking.

High-Oleic Canola Oil: 1 serving = 1 tablespoon

High-oleic canola oil can be used as a substitute for regular vegetable oil in baking in any situation where extra-virgin olive oil would not be appropriate (for example, olive oil might ruin the flavor of a fruit muffin or other baked good). High-oleic canola oil contains less than half as much essential fat as you would find in regular expeller-pressed canola oil. Consequently, high-oleic canola oil is much more heat-stable and better for cooking than regular canola oil.

High-oleic canola oils typically say either "high-oleic" or "safe for high-heat cooking" or "super" on their labeling. Note, however, the statement "safe for high-heat cooking" is not regulated and does not absolutely guarantee that the product is high-oleic. To be sure, read the back of the nutrition label and look under the total fat content; high-oleic oils should contain just 2 grams of polyunsaturated fat per tablespoon. Unless you are 100 percent sure, stick to brands that specifically say "high-oleic" on the package label. One brand we recommend that is easy to locate in the natural foods store is Spectrum Natural's Super Canola Oil. Also, when purchasing prepackaged foods that you intend to heat or that have already been heated during processing, be sure to look for the words "high-oleic" on the label.

"With Mayo, Please"

Mayonnaise made from canola oil is a delicious alternative to conventional mayonnaise, a product that is often loaded with excess amounts of low-quality omega-6 vegetable oil. Canola oil mayonnaise is available at any natural foods store and is a healthy, delicious spread alternative for those of you who love mayonnaise.

High-Oleic Sunflower Oil and High-Oleic Safflower Oil:

1 serving = 1 tablespoon

Both high-oleic sunflower oil and high-oleic safflower oil can be used for cooking and baking just like high-oleic canola oil. Use these oils instead of vegetable oils in cooking and baking whenever extra-virgin olive oil would not be appropriate. Spectrum Naturals is a high-quality brand name you can trust as a source for high-oleic sunflower and safflower oils.

Eat High-Oleic Oils in Moderation

Keep in mind that although we do allow high-oleic canola oil, sun-flower oil and safflower oil as part of the Cure, you should use these oils in moderation. They are not as nutrient-rich as extra-virgin olive oil, and they contain far less omega-3 fat than either expeller-pressed canola oil or flax oil. While they won't harm your health, they haven't been clinically proven to enhance your health either. Think of these oils as being neutral as opposed to wonderful.

Nuts: 1 serving = 2 heaping tablespoons

Nuts, as long as they have *not* been roasted in the vegetable oils you are trying to avoid, are a wonderfully healthful whole foods choice. Buy either dry-roasted nuts or raw nuts. Most nuts are rich in healthful monounsaturated fat as well as all-natural, undamaged, essential omega-6 fat. Nuts contain vitamins and minerals, includ-ing large amounts of heart-healthy magnesium, fiber, protein and antioxidants—and some even contain omega-3 fat.

Numerous studies in well-esteemed medical journals have reported major cardiovascular benefits associated with eating nuts regularly. In the July 2001 issue of the *American Journal of Clinical Nutrition,* researchers documented that walnuts could reduce total cholesterol level, and bad cholesterol level, even when no other dietary changes were made.[4] Macadamia nuts have been shown to produce similar benefits,[5] and pecans have also been shown to be beneficial.[6]

Nuts offer more than just cardiovascular benefits. Nuts, and all-natural nut butters such as peanut butter, have been shown to reduce your risk of developing diabetes[7] and provide protection against colon cancer. If you avoid nuts because you think they're fattening, studies show people who are allowed to eat as many nuts as they like on a regular basis are actually slimmer than those who don't eat nuts.[8] Harvard researchers recently concluded that the evidence supporting increased nut consumption is strong enough to warrant modification of the U.S. government's official "food pyramid."[9] The bottom line when it comes to these studies is that the type of nut you choose to eat does *not* matter. All nuts are healthful as long as they're not roasted in oil.

All-Natural Nut Butters: 1 serving = 1 tablespoon

Everything good about nuts also applies to nut butters. These are healthful foods with one big caveat: In order to obtain the health benefits from eating nut butters you must purchase "all-natural" products. When purchasing any type of nut butter read the label very carefully. The product you choose must contain absolutely no hydrogenated oils, absolutely no partially hydrogenated oils and absolutely no added sugar. The list of ingredients should say only "nuts" and maybe "salt." No other ingredients are needed to make nut butter. Nut butters that meet these requirements almost always specifically advertise themselves as being all-natural. Natural food stores tend to have a better selection of all-natural nut butters than the average supermarket. While peanut butter is great, try other equally healthful, more exotic nut butters such as almond butter, cashew nut butter and hazelnut butter.

Avocado: 1 serving = ¼ of a medium-sized avocado

The avocado is brimming with heart-healthy nutrients. Avocados contain vitamin E, folate, vitamin C, potassium, the phytochemical alpha-carotene and monounsaturated fat. This nutritional powerhouse does wonders for improving the health and appearance of your skin, too. If you think avocados are fattening, rest assured: They don't contribute to weight gain. Avocados actually depress insulin production and help keep you feeling full and satisfied long after mealtime, a great formula for weight management.

Avocado Oil: 1 serving = 1 tablespoon

Because avocado oil is rich in heat-stable monounsaturated fat, it's safe for cooking. Many gourmet chefs like the full-bodied, slightly nutty flavor of this oil and use it in a variety of both cold and warm dishes. For variety, try substituting avocado oil for olive oil in vegetable dishes, bean dips, chicken recipes and so forth.

BOTTOM LINE ————————————————————————————

All monounsaturated fats are acceptable on the *Cure*.

The Cheat Sheet on Monounsaturated Fats and Oils

- Extra-virgin olive oil is the best oil for cooking because it's extremely heat stable. While extra-virgin olive oil is also good for no-heat recipes, we recommend you use flax oil as much as possible in this situation. Extra-virgin olive oil is always a good choice when dining out.
- Include at least one or two foods high in monounsaturated fat as part of your diet every day. Nuts, nut butters and avocados are excellent.
- Use high-oleic canola oil, high-oleic safflower oil and high-oleic sunflower oil in moderation when you prepare recipes requiring heat. Limit your use of these oils to those few recipes that just wouldn't taste right if you used extra-virgin olive oil. While extra-virgin olive oil is best, all of these alternative high-oleic oils are much better for your health than standard vegetable oil.
- High-quality expeller-pressed canola oil is acceptable for use in no-heat recipes, but flax oil is always a better choice.

Now that you know more about how some oils can better your health, chapter 6 introduces two super foods no diet should be without.

Two Power Proteins: Fish and Soy

6

You'll notice that we've spent very little time in this book talking about protein. The truth is, the typical American eats way too much protein, and protein isn't a "free food." Your body needs only about a half a gram of protein per pound of body weight—any excess amounts to empty calories. In fact, the December 2001 *Tufts University Health & Nutrition Letter* reported that the American Heart Association, the American College of Sports Medicine, the Cooper Institute for Aerobics Research and the Women's Sports Foundation take the position that high-protein diets are not healthy.[1] Rest assured, the Gold Coast Cure is not a high-protein diet.

To enjoy optimal health you need to eat either fish or soy *every single day*. This is not hard to do if you make a conscious effort to make one of them the main protein source for one of your daily meals. You can still enjoy chicken, eggs, milk, meat, cheese, turkey or any other protein food for your other two meals or as snacks. For example, if you're going to a steakhouse Monday night for filet mignon, then eat vegetarian chili made with soybeans or grilled fish for lunch. If on Tuesday you eat a tuna wrap for lunch, you could have a chicken and cheese burrito for dinner. If on Wednesday you eat a cheese omelet for breakfast, try a veggie burger made from soy for lunch. If on Thursday you have a soy-strawberry smoothie for breakfast, then go ahead and enjoy pork tenderloin for dinner. If you particularly like fish and soy, it's perfectly fine to eat them more than once a day.

Why Fish?

All fish (including shellfish) are healthful and contain a high percentage of omega-3 fat when compared to other commonly eaten foods. However, certain fatty species of fish provide the maximum possible health benefit because they contain the most omega-3 fat. Don't be put off by the word "fatty"; these fish contain very little bad fat. In general, the fattiest, most healthful fish tend to be cold water species. Please refer to Table 6.1.

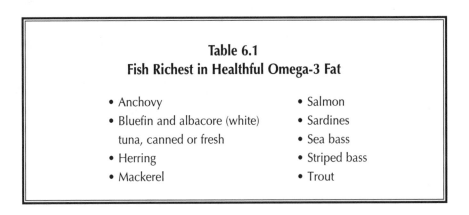

Table 6.1
Fish Richest in Healthful Omega-3 Fat

- Anchovy
- Bluefin and albacore (white) tuna, canned or fresh
- Herring
- Mackerel
- Salmon
- Sardines
- Sea bass
- Striped bass
- Trout

It doesn't matter whether you eat farmed or wild fish. From a health standpoint, you should concentrate more on preparing fish healthfully, without frying, and less on where they are caught. Canned fish and smoked fish are good, too, as long as you purchase canned fish that's packed in water or olive oil instead of soybean oil or other vegetable oils.

Despite the health benefits of fish, be careful how you prepare it. Fish that's breaded with empty-calorie refined flour, then deep-fried in unhealthful oil is almost as bad as eating a bag of chips. If you serve fish with tartar sauce made from refined vegetable oil or drown your fish in a fat-laden cream sauce, you cancel out the health benefits. An academic study recently published in a prestigious journal backs this up. Researchers showed *no* health benefit associated with eating fish when the fish was prepared in an unhealthy manner, but this same study showed a 50 percent decrease in death due to heart disease among persons who ate healthfully prepared fish three or more times per week.[2]

Although there's conflicting information about how much fish you need to eat, most health organizations and nutritionists agree that fish should be an integral part of your diet. The American Heart Association recommends eating at least two servings of fish every week. At a 1999 National Institutes of Health conference, a consensus was reached that a total of 3 grams of the omega-3 fats EPA and DHA, the amount contained in about half a pound of fatty fish, should be eaten *every* day for optimal health.

Let's be realistic, though: Eating half a pound of fatty fish daily is not practical. We try to eat fish for lunch or dinner at least four times a week at least two of these meals include fatty fish, bringing us close to the optimal level of EPA and DHA intake based solely upon our diets. If you can't eat this much fish, you can take fish oil supplements, as detailed in chapter 11. And remember, every bit of fish you eat is helpful.

Fish and Your Health

If you're not too keen on fish, you may be when you check out its inherent health benefits.

It's Good for Your Heart

A number of studies published in some of the very best medical journals have repeatedly proven that eating fish regularly can prevent, reverse and even cure cardiovascular conditions, including atherosclerosis,[3] cardiac arrhythmias, stroke,[4] peripheral vascular disease, high blood pressure[5] and even sudden cardiac death.[6]

A diet rich in foods containing EPA and DHA can reduce your triglyceride level by up to 65 percent. In fact, no dietary therapy is more effective at reducing your blood triglyceride level than eating fatty fish. Even if your doctor prescribes medicine you should still eat fish. The triglyceride-lowering effects you get from eating the omega-3 fats found in fish are in addition to any triglyceride-lowering effects you get from taking medications.[7]

It's Good for Diabetics and People with Prediabetes

The omega-3 fats in fish are especially helpful for diabetics and pre-diabetics. Diabetes and prediabetes significantly increase your risk of developing heart disease. The essential fats in fish oil have been proven to improve your blood lipid profile, decrease platelet aggregation, decrease triglycerides and decrease blood pressure. All four of these health improvements greatly reduce your risk of heart disease whether or not you are diabetic. What's more, fish oils protect against diabetic neuropathy,[8] a debilitating, painful complication of diabetes that often leads to amputation.

In a sixteen-year study involving more than five thousand diabetic women, increased fish intake reduced their total death rate by over 50 percent.[9]

Diabetics should be aware that fatty fish and fish oil supplementation can have an unpredictable effect on their blood sugar level. Some studies have shown a worsening of blood sugar control in the weeks following increased intake of fish and fish oil. Sure enough, some of our clients have reported elevations in their blood glucose level following intake of fish oil supplements. This is probably due to the fact that fish oil prevents insulin from converting glucose into triglycerides. This conversion normally occurs whenever too many empty carbohydrates are eaten too quickly. In diabetics, if glucose cannot be converted into triglycerides, the excess blood sugar has nowhere else to go, at least in the short term. The diabetic's blood sugar level may therefore *temporarily* stay higher than usual.

This is not a problem. Because your triglyceride levels drop significantly, the net effect is positive even if your blood sugar level does go up for a little while. Studies show there are no long-term problems with glucose tolerance following supplementation with omega-3 fat.[10] One study showed that *if* there is an increase in your blood sugar level, it can be completely reversed by adding exercise to your total lifestyle regimen.[11] And, if you're following the Cure in its entirety, you should be performing thirty minutes of exercise three times a week anyway.

Eating fish for the sake of improving the diabetic person's overall health is not at all controversial: Diabetics should follow the same lifestyle recommendations we make to all people in the Gold Coast Cure.

It Can Help Protect Against Cancer

Increasingly irrefutable evidence shows that diets rich in omega-3 fats offer significant protection against cancer. Fish is rich in iodine, a mineral required for the prevention of many thyroid conditions, and it has been shown to help reduce your risk of developing thyroid cancer, especially if you happen to live in an iodine-deficient region.[12] People who consume fish on a regular basis have also been reported to have low risks of cancers of the pancreas, colon[13] and prostate.[14]

It's Good for Inflammatory Conditions

DHA and EPA help your body increase its production of several inflammation fighters and a host of other important anti-inflammatory hormones that reduce the symptoms of many inflammatory conditions. While the evidence is stronger for some conditions than it is for others, this largely has to do with the amount of effort scientists have spent studying each individual condition. These include:

- Allergies
- Chronic obstructive pulmonary disease
- Crohn's disease
- Vascular dementia and Alzheimer's disease[15]
- Psoriasis
- Asthma
- Exercise-induced asthma[16]
- Multiple sclerosis[17, 18]
- Rheumatoid arthritis[19]
- Ulcerative colitis[20]
- Fibromyalgia
- Osteoarthritis

Getting Kids to Eat Their Fish

Children, especially, benefit from eating fish. Their growing brains—even prior to birth—benefit from EPA and DHA. A randomized, double-blind study reported in the prestigious journal *Pediatrics* recently showed that fortification of mother's diet during the second half of pregnancy and during the first three months of lactation with the EPA and DHA in cod liver oil resulted in improved childhood intelligence at age four.[21] Brains grow most rapidly during the first few months of life. Research shows infants who are even mildly deficient in DHA attain less than optimal neural development and are at risk for lowered intelligence and less than optimal vision.

In 1996, researchers at Purdue University found that boys with low levels of omega-3 fat in their blood displayed more problems with behavior, more learning difficulties and more health problems compared with boys who had higher blood levels of omega-3 fat.[22]

While decades ago children didn't suffer from "adult diseases," that's not the case today. Unfortunately, kids today are suffering from type II diabetes, high cholesterol levels and obesity, and some of the same inflammatory conditions as adults, all of which can be helped by a diet rich in fish. Childhood asthma and allergies are more common today than they have ever been, and fish and fish oil supplements can significantly ameliorate childhood asthma symptoms.[23] Fish might even reduce your child's need to take asthma medication, especially if you reduce your child's intake of saturated fats and trans fats. Infants born to mothers who supplement with omega-3 fat during pregnancy are less likely to develop food allergies and develop less severe cases of dermatitis.[24] The bottom line is kids need to eat fish, too.

The Mercury Scare: Is It Justified?

Unfortunately, despite an overwhelming amount of research documenting massive health benefits associated with increased consumption of fish and fish oil, many people are hung up worrying about the possibility that the organic mercury found within certain species of fish is harmful to their health. We strongly believe this concern is complete nonsense, based on studies demonstrating the positive effects of eating fish, including heart benefits, decreased depression, decreased Alzheimer's disease and more.

We know there is mercury in fish, and we know that mercury can be poisonous. We acknowledge also that people who eat fish have higher blood mercury levels than people who do not.[25] More important, however, we know multiple studies have been done on real people in real life that have proven beyond a shadow of doubt that fish eaters *live longer* and suffer fewer heart attacks than people who do not eat fish.[26] To us, the prevailing issue is not mercury levels in the blood but long life and optimal health. The people who got mercury poisoning back in the nineteenth century worked in factories where huge concentrations of mercury were present and safety regulations were nonexistent. They did not get mercury poisoning from eating fish.

We would rather you eat fish and enjoy a proven 50 percent reduction in your risk of heart attack. The same advice goes for children. There is no known association between daily fish consumption and problems with childhood development. As a matter of fact, the largest scientific study performed to date has specifically shown there to be no harmful relationship between either prenatal or postnatal mercury exposure and developmental outcomes in either five-year-olds[27] or nine-year-olds.[28] In these studies, childbearing women ate on average twelve servings of fish *weekly*.

If you're pregnant or the parent of a young child and you're still concerned, high-quality fish oil supplementation is a perfectly viable alternative to eating fish. Commercially available fish oil pills are made primarily from species such as cod, herring, sardines, menhaden and anchovy that have not been implicated as sources of mercury. These pills have been proven to contain no more mercury than is naturally present in the human bloodstream.[29] We recommend that anyone concerned about potential mercury dangers at least take the fish oil supplements we recommend; it's almost impossible to obtain optimal amounts of the omega-3 fats DHA and EPA otherwise.

In our opinion, certain misguided organizations have been overly conservative in their recommendations, especially since there is no reliable evidence proving that eating the small amount of mercury found in fish is associated with risk to adults or children. The government has been wrong before, especially when it comes to telling us what we should or should not be putting into our mouths. The government was behind the low-fat movement and supported the ill-conceived switch from butter to margarine.

We've read the relevant research and see no reason to fear the mercury in fish. If you're still concerned, the Center for Food Safety and Applied Nutrition maintains a table listing mean mercury levels for many fish species at *www.cfsan.fda.gov/~frf/sea-mehg.html*. It's been well-publicized that tilefish, shark, swordfish and king mackerel contain the highest concentrations of organic mercury on the average, so you can avoid eating these kinds of fish if you're concerned. Most of the fatty fish we recommend, including salmon, trout, herring, sardines and anchovy, contain very low levels of mercury on the average.

BOTTOM LINE ————————————————————————————————

Eat at least two servings of fatty fish every week, and try to eat at least four total servings of any kind of fish every week.

As parents ourselves we realize getting your children to eat fish can be about as easy as getting them to go to bed willingly or sit quietly for more than ten minutes at a time. There is a solution: your children can obtain the same benefits from fish oil supplementation as they would from eating fish, without you worrying about mercury poisoning or having to hear your child complain about the "yuckies."

For children, we recommend Nordic Naturals ProEFA Liquid, an omega-3 fish oil supplement that also contains GLA, a good omega-6 fat that many children are deficient in. Children under fifty pounds should take ¼ teaspoon daily, and children over fifty pounds should take ½ teaspoon daily. Adults can take this supplement, too, although we recommend the higher-dosage Ultimate Omega brand of omega-3 fat supplement in combination with the GLA found in evening primrose oil (see chapter 11 for more details) for adults who are able to swallow pills. You can learn more about Nordic Naturals by visiting their Web site at *www.nordicnaturals.com*. Their products may be ordered online if they are not available at your local health food store.

Just Say Soy

Soy is a true super-food that's been associated with health, vitality and longevity for centuries. Although whole soy has been an important food source for over five thousand years in many East Asian cultures, it's only now enjoying appropriate mainstream interest in the West.

The Joy of Soy

1) **Soybeans are a nutrient-rich whole food.**

Soy is the *only* vegetarian source of complete protein. The World Health Organization has established that soy protein eaten alone, even if no other complementary foods are eaten, contains high enough concentrations of all the essential amino acids necessary to meet human requirements so long as soy protein is consumed at the recommended level of daily protein intake.[30] In addition to being protein-rich, soy is also a good source of essential fat and important micronutrients such as calcium, vitamin B_{12} and iron.

2) **Soy is low in saturated fat.**

Soy is a superb alternative to animal protein, providing your body with the complete protein found in animal foods without the negatives associated with eating too much saturated fat. If you have heart disease, diabetes or any inflammation-mediated condition such as multiple sclerosis, asthma, arthritis or fibromyalgia, replacing saturated fat–rich animal protein with soy protein is especially beneficial.

3) **Soy contains essential fat.**

Fifty percent of the fat in the soybean is omega-6 fat while 7 percent of the fat in soybeans is omega-3 fat. Of the commonly available vegetarian foods, only canola oil, walnuts and flax contain a greater percentage of omega-3 fat than soy. The omega-6 essential fat found in whole soy foods (but not processed soybean oil) is the healthful, unrefined, unheated type of omega-6 fat you do need to eat more of. Eating soy regularly helps ensure you get both omega-3 and omega-6 essential fats.

4) **Soy protects your heart.**

Soy protects your entire cardiovascular system by altering your cholesterol profile for the better. In human studies, soy has been proven to lower bad LDL cholesterol levels, decrease overall cholesterol absorption and increase cholesterol excretion. The American Heart Association states, "There is increasing evidence that the consumption of soy protein may help lower blood cholesterol levels in some people with elevated total cholesterol levels, and may provide other cardiovascular benefits."[31] In the *New England Journal of Medicine,* one of the most respected journals in medicine, researchers report, ". . . the consumption of soy protein rather than animal protein significantly decreased serum concentrations of total cholesterol, LDL cholesterol, and triglycerides."[32]

Since 1999 the U.S. Food and Drug Administration has allowed soy food manufacturers to make advertising claims stating "diets rich in soy protein and low in saturated fat can reduce the risk of coronary heart disease." Replacing some of the animal protein foods you currently eat with soy is an effective way to reduce your overall saturated fat intake without decreasing your protein intake. The end result is significantly improved cardiovascular health.

5) **Soy can help you stay slim.**

Soy is a nutrient-dense food providing lots of satiety in a low-calorie package. Because it's slowly digested, it has a minimal effect on blood sugar and insulin levels. Many soy foods, such as soybeans and soy burgers, also contain fiber and are especially filling.

6) **Soy contains health-preserving, health-enhancing phytochemicals.**

Phytochemicals are nonvitamin substances found in plant foods that possess disease-preventing qualities. Scientific evidence proves phytochemicals help prevent and treat at least four leading causes of premature death, namely cancer, diabetes, hypertension and cardiovascular disease.[33]

7) **Soy is one of the richest food sources of health-promoting phytoestrogens.**

Phytoestrogens are natural plant compounds capable of exerting mild estrogen-like actions in the body, which benefit women and men. Phytoestrogens partially inhibit the activity of excess human estrogens, and studies suggest soy foods have a beneficial role in protecting against hormone-sensitive cancers such as breast and prostate cancer as well as osteoporosis and menopausal symptoms.

The phytoestrogens in soy are thought to be natural selective estrogen receptor modulators, also referred to as SERMs. Other SERMs you may have read about include tamoxifen, a powerful medicine used to treat breast cancer, and raloxifene, a drug used to slow the effects of osteoporosis. The phytochemicals in soy possess many desirable SERM effects without causing side effects like hot flashes, blood clots and uterine cancer.

Ladies First ...

Soy phytoestrogens are especially helpful for adult women because they're a natural alternative to hormone replacement therapy during menopause. Although a variety of theoretical explanations exist, scientists believe the phytoestrogens found in soy to some extent mimic the effects of natural estrogens. In countries where soy is consumed regularly, women experience far fewer bothersome menopausal symptoms when compared with women in countries where soy is eaten infrequently. Japanese women who consume more soy products are significantly less likely to develop menopausal hot flashes.[34]

Phytoestrogen Supplements Don't Work

Please note that many studies show minimal to no benefit from taking isolated phytoestrogens in pill form. Therefore, we strongly recommend eating only whole soy foods instead of isolated phytoestrogen supplements.

Women are especially prone to osteoporosis. Through a combination of mechanisms, whole soy foods also provide protection against osteoporosis. In 2000 the *American Journal of Clinical Nutrition* reported soy intake can reduce the loss of bone in the lower back commonly associated with menopause.[35] While the phytoestrogens in soy play an important role in bone protection, the combination of minerals and nutrients found in whole soy foods helps, too. Although calcium is quite popular for its protective effect on our bones, many people are unaware that magnesium is essential for the transport of calcium from the bloodstream to the bones. In other words, without an adequate intake of magnesium, calcium is not nearly as beneficial. Unlike other calcium-rich foods such as dairy products, soy is rich in both calcium *and* magnesium.

Soy helps prevent excess estrogens in your body from inappropriately activating your estrogen receptors. Excess estrogens in your body increase your risk of acquiring hormone-sensitive cancers such as breast cancer. It is not commonly known, but your body's fat cells produce "natural" estrogens that can also increase your chance of breast cancer. For this very reason, obese women have approximately twice the risk of acquiring breast cancer as women of normal weight. This relationship is especially noticeable in postmenopausal women.[36] Soy can help reduce your risk of hormone-sensitive cancers by taking up parking space in your body's estrogen receptors without fully activating these receptors. The phytoestrogens in soy have the ability to block out the toxic effects of those excess "natural" estrogens floating around in your bloodstream.

Population-based studies supporting soy's role in cancer prevention are especially intriguing. In one study, over fourteen hundred Chinese women who had been diagnosed with breast cancer were compared with more than fifteen hundred age-matched women without breast cancer. These researchers showed that high levels of soy intake were associated with a significantly reduced chance of being diagnosed with breast cancer.[37]

Important Information for Breast Cancer Patients

While phytoestrogens protect against the *development* of breast cancer[38] they may interfere with the action of certain drugs used to *treat* breast cancer. Drugs such as tamoxifen and raloxifene are very powerful selective estrogen receptor modulators (SERMs). People who have *already* been diagnosed with breast cancer need to take the most powerful treatment available despite any negative side effects associated with it. Because phytoestrogens may take up space on the same receptors that would be blocked by cancer-fighting drugs such as tamoxifen, it's best not to eat large amounts of soy if you're under active treatment for breast cancer with tamoxifen or raloxifene. The same logic would apply to taking isoflavone supplements in pill form. We recommend you consult your doctor about food choices during treatment for any type of cancer.

Real Men Do Eat Tofu

The phytoestrogens in soy offer protection against prostate cancer, the third most deadly cancer in men. Two hundred thousand American men—more men than live in either Orlando, Florida, or Buffalo, New York—are diagnosed with prostate cancer every year. According to the American Cancer Society, thirty thousand of them will die from the disease in any given year. It's tragic that while men are smoking less and trying to take better care of their hearts, they are ignoring preventive maintenance on their prostate glands. This is especially unfortunate because prostate cancer is one of the most preventable cancers.

In East Asian countries where soy is a dietary staple, prostate cancer mortality is significantly lower than it is in the United States. In Japan, prostate cancer mortality is only 30 percent as high as it is in the United

States even though Japanese men live longer than American men. Two large population-based studies show less prostate cancer in men who eat more soy products.[39, 40] Researchers have concluded that the consumption of soy products is more protective against prostate cancer than any other known dietary factor. It's unfortunate that no prospective, randomized clinical trials of high quality have explored this low-cost way to protect men against this extremely common cancer.

Where Can I Find Whole Soy?

In most places you won't need to schlep to some out-of-the-way store to find soy. You can find most of the thirteen whole soy foods we recommend below at your local supermarket:

1) **Tofu.** Tofu has a neutral flavor, and it makes a great accompaniment to strongly flavored sauces. "Soft" and "silken" tofu blends well into shakes, puddings and soups. "Firm" or "extra firm" tofu patties are wonderful as an entrée when they are grilled or stir-fried (in good oils, of course) then topped with your favorite sauce.
2) **Miso.** Miso is great in soups and stews.
3) **Natto.** A Japanese staple made by fermenting soybeans.
4) **Soybeans.** Salted and dry-roasted soybeans are readily available in grocery stores and are perfect for on-the-go snacking. Natural foods stores also sell raw soybeans and canned soybeans in a variety of flavors.
5) **Edamame beans.** These delicious, edible soybeans were initially popularized in Japanese restaurants and are a great way to introduce soy into your child's diet; our son goes crazy for them.
6) **Tempeh.** This Indonesian favorite has a firm texture, chewy consistency and nutty, mushroom-like flavor. It's great on the grill and can also be sautéed in extra-virgin olive oil or a little melted butter.

7) **Soy milk.** You can drink regular or sweetened soy milk. The leading brand of sweetened soy milk contains only about twenty calories' worth of added sugar per serving.

8) **Soy flour.** Avoid "de-fatted" soy flours because the fat in soy is healthful, filling and essential.

9) **Soy cheese.** Low in saturated fat and an excellent alternative to dairy cheese, soy cheese contains calcium and magnesium.

10) **Soy burgers.** Be sure the brand you purchase does not contain hydrogenated oils or partially hydrogenated oils, otherwise you will lose all the health benefits you hope to gain by eating soy burgers in the first place.

11) **Soy chili.** A wide variety of vegetarian, soy-based, canned chili is available at your local natural foods store. Experiment to find the best-tasting brand. We like to mix canned soups and canned chili with fresh ingredients, such as additional vege-tables and garlic, for a more homemade taste.

12) **Soy protein shakes.** We like the Spirutein brand best. Soy protein shakes can be blended with fruit, flaxseeds, and soy milk or low-fat milk for a quick and easy breakfast.

13) **Textured soy protein.** Soy protein can be used as a meat substitute in any dish that calls for ground meat. You can also mix it with ground beef or ground turkey to make meatballs or meat loaf that has both the flavor of meat and the health benefits of soy.

One Soy Product to Avoid

Although soybean oil is made from whole soybeans, soybean oil is *not* a Gold Coast Cure–approved food. Extra-virgin olive oil, high-quality expeller-pressed canola oil (for no-heat recipes), flax oil, high-oleic canola oil, high-oleic safflower oil and high-oleic sunflower oil are all much better choices. Even butter is healthier than grocery store soybean oil.

Commercial soybean oil is a highly refined, heat-damaged product that you should avoid at all costs. Refined oils undergo degumming, bleaching and deodorizing processes that remove nutrients while adding free radicals and other byproducts of oxidation. The essential fats in soybeans are changed and destroyed when refined into oil. Soybean oil contains no phytoestrogens, no magnesium, no vitamins and no other nutrients of any kind. In other words, it's an empty-calorie food.

BOTTOM LINE —————————————————————————
Eat soy or fish every single day.

In Conclusion

Soy and fish are not "magic bullets" for optimal health. We all know that if we eat Big Macs for lunch every day and then go home and take a fish pill with our dinner or have a soy milk shake for dessert we can't expect glowing health. However, an overwhelming amount of research shows that if you make the effort to substitute a few less healthful foods for soy and fish, you will *substantially* improve your overall health, you will live longer and you will feel better—even if you happen to cheat a little bit.

Now that you know you should try to add fish and soy to your diet, let's move on to what you can drink on the Cure.

A Toast to Your Health: What You Can Drink on the Cure

We all know that water is healthful; however, there's no need to obsess over exactly how much water you drink. Just be sure to drink water whenever you're thirsty. Calorie-free beverages such as seltzer water are acceptable substitutes for water.

Is Alcohol Allowed on the Cure?

It goes without saying that if you drink too much alcohol, you will seriously harm your health and appearance and possibly the health of others. However, overwhelming scientific evidence shows that alcohol, when consumed at the right amounts, has the potential to enhance your health and well-being. Therefore, alcohol, especially wine, is acceptable in *moderation* as part of the Gold Coast Cure.

Studies in the medical literature such as the Copenhagen City Heart Study[1] and the Framingham Heart Study[2] have found that consuming wine in *moderation* is associated with an increased life expectancy.

Moderation means no more than 1½ drinks per day for women and no more than 2½ drinks per day for men. One drink is equivalent to one 12-ounce beer, one 5-ounce glass of wine, or one shot (1½ ounces) of hard alcohol. One standard bottle of wine contains five glasses of wine. The "big" bottles of wine contain ten glasses.

The quantities above should be considered maximum daily intake. Optimal intake is slightly less, probably just under one drink per day for women and just under two drinks per day for men.

Most studies show the first one or two drinks *per week* are by far the most beneficial, so there is no need to drink alcohol every night of the week. If you're not in the habit of drinking alcohol, consider enjoying one glass of wine with dinner once or twice a week and leaving it at that.

Although population surveys show moderate drinkers are healthier than teetotalers, there is no reason to start drinking if you don't already. Alcohol is optional on the Gold Coast Cure. You can dramatically improve your health and dramatically reduce your risk of early death by following our whole foods diet and sticking to the nutritional supplementation regimen and resistance circuit training exercises we teach in our later chapters. You do not need to take a single sip of alcohol to enjoy good health.

This having been said, those of you who avoid alcohol for health reasons need to seriously consider the science. We have come across many wellness books and many weight-loss books that recommend no alcohol consumption without providing any scientific rationale. These books are just plain wrong. Moderate consumption of alcohol as part of an otherwise healthful lifestyle causes no negative health consequences and, for most people, provides significant health benefits.

Here's to Your Health

In a sixteen-year study examining data from the Copenhagen City Heart Study, researchers found intake of wine (but not beer or liquor) on either a monthly, weekly or daily basis was associated with a lower risk of stroke as compared with not consuming wine at all. Dr. Thomas

Truelsen and colleagues concluded, "Whatever the biological mechanism may be, the consistency of the results, the lack of obvious biases, and the biological plausibility suggest that there may be a beneficial effect of intake of wine on risk of stroke."[3] This decreased risk of stroke was confirmed in the United States in the Northern Manhattan Stroke study. Researchers examined alcohol consumption in more than eighteen hundred Manhattan men and women. They found a nearly 50 percent decrease in the risk of stroke for men and women who consumed up to two drinks per day.[4]

While it seems almost counterintuitive to think that wine can protect your mental faculties, according to research published in the *Journal of the American Medical Association*, moderate drinkers have a decreased risk of developing Alzheimer's disease when compared with nondrinkers.[5] This study confirmed what had already been shown in two large European studies.[6,7] Most senility is caused at least in part by vascular disease. Wine appears to keep your arteries clean and your thinking clear.

Can Diabetics Propose a Toast?

Moderate alcohol intake has been associated with a reduced fasting insulin concentration, improved insulin sensitivity and a reduced risk for developing diabetes. Alcohol drinkers have lower insulin levels compared with nondrinkers consuming the same amount of calories.[8] In the Nurses' Health Study, drinkers were at significantly less risk for developing diabetes as compared with teetotalers.[9] Furthermore, people who already have diabetes are less likely to develop heart disease if they drink alcohol.[10] There is no reason for the diabetic to avoid alcohol.

Weighing In

Here comes the big question: Will moderate drinking make you fat? The evidence indicates the answer is no. In April 1997, the *Journal of the American College of Nutrition* reported on a twelve-week crossover study. Fourteen men were given two glasses of wine to drink every day for six weeks, and then they were asked to abstain for six weeks. The men did not gain weight while they were drinking nor did they lose weight upon stopping. They were allowed to eat whatever else they desired throughout the study period.[11] Two glasses of wine contain about two hundred calories. Over a six-week period these men should have gained about two and a half pounds, yet they did not.

A more recent study showed that women who routinely drank moderate amounts of alcohol, adding up to about one drink per day, carried almost ten pounds less body fat than women who did not drink at all.[12] Prior to this, researchers at the Centers for Disease Control showed that, over a ten-year study period, drinking alcohol seemed to have very little effect on body weight. In this study drinkers tended to gain less weight when compared with people who abstained from alcohol.[13] In a similar ten-year study, drinkers displayed a slight tendency to *lose* weight.[14]

While no one really knows for sure why the calories in alcohol do not appear to be metabolized in the same manner as the calories from carbohydrates, fats and protein, there is no scientific rationale to abstain from drinking moderate amounts of alcohol just because you are trying to lose weight.

The Most Healthful Alcohol

Several large-scale population studies show wine drinkers are healthier than either beer drinkers or hard liquor drinkers. In the landmark 1995 Copenhagen City Heart Study, one of the first studies to look at this question specifically, low to moderate intake of wine was associated with a lower mortality from cardiovascular disease, stroke, and all other causes as compared to abstainers and as compared with drinkers who consumed other types of alcohol.[15] Compared with abstainers, wine drinkers had a 50 percent reduced risk of *death* over the course of the twelve-year study, while beer drinkers received no benefit and hard alcohol drinkers actually had an *increased* risk of dying.

It's fair to mention that other studies have not necessarily come to the same conclusion. A recent study in the *New England Journal of Medicine* showed men who drank alcohol three to seven days out of the week had far fewer heart attacks than men who drank less than once per week. These researchers failed to identify any difference based upon the type of alcohol consumed, be it wine, beer or hard liquor.[16] This study is in the minority; most medical literature shows that wine is better for you than beer and beer is better for you than hard alcohol.

When it comes to choosing red or white wine, those of you who read frequently about health may have developed a bias in favor of red. Resveratrol and quercetin are two antioxidants found in red wine that are lacking in white wine. This doesn't mean white wine is no good; it offers its own unique set of antioxidants. No proof exists that resveratrol and quercetin provide health benefits greater than those provided by other antioxidants. A recent U.S. study involving more than one hundred thousand people confirmed that wine drinkers were significantly less likely to die over the twenty-year study period as compared with persons who favored beer or hard alcohol.[17] These researchers looked carefully but they were unable to detect any difference in mortality based upon whether white wine, red wine or any other type of wine was the beverage of choice. Wine contains antioxidants, and it's very low in sugar. Even sweet dessert wines are relatively low in sugar when compared with most alternative beverages.

Beer also contains antioxidants but it contains more sugar carbohydrates than wine. The empty-calorie sugar carbohydrates in beer cancel out most of the health-providing effects of the alcohol and antioxidants. While light beers contain less sugar than darker beers, they also contain fewer antioxidants. Hard liquor served straight up doesn't contain sugar, but it also doesn't have any antioxidants. Even worse, people often mix hard liquor with sugary soft drinks, high-calorie juices, sugar syrups and even saturated fat–rich creams. It's not surprising, then, that most studies show wine to be the most healthful alcoholic beverage, regardless of its color.

Beer and hard liquor are acceptable to drink a few times a month. When drinking hard liquor, don't sweeten it with high-sugar, non-natural additives. For example, despite its dry flavor, tonic water contains lots of added sugar.

BOTTOM LINE ————————————————————————
Women can consume 5 ounces of wine up to seven days a week. Men can consume 10 ounces of wine up to seven days a week. Beer and hard liquor may be enjoyed instead of wine two or three times a month.

Coffee

Coffee is not as unhealthful as some diet books would like you to believe. As a matter of fact, high-quality research links coffee with numerous health *benefits*.

Coffee beans are loaded with antioxidants, some of which become even more potent during the roasting process. Antioxidants protect against oxidative stress by "mopping up" damaging free radicals that have been implicated in cancer, heart disease and the aging process in general. The latest scientific evidence indicates drinking two to four cups of coffee per day is not harmful and may even provide significant health benefits. In a Japanese study, coffee consumption was associated with a decreased risk of death from *all* causes.[18]

A Cup of Joe May Reduce Your Risk of Diabetes

Coffee may also provide protection against diabetes. Researchers at the Harvard School of Public Health and the Brigham and Women's Hospital found study subjects who regularly drank coffee had a significantly reduced risk of developing diabetes over a twelve- to eighteen-year study period as compared to people who didn't drink coffee.[19] Another study reported in the *Journal of the American Medical Association* examined more than 14,600 people from Finland.[20] Researchers discovered that Finnish women and men who drank three to four cups of coffee daily had a greater than 25 percent reduced risk of developing diabetes. Be sure your coffee doesn't contain empty-calorie sugar or too much cream, and most definitely do not add nondairy powdered creamer that contains trans fat.

The Parkinson's Paradox

Can coffee, a substance known to cause the jitters, actually help prevent a disease characterized by tremors? While it sounds ridiculous, research shows it's true. The *Journal of the American Medical Association* published the results of a study examining 8,004 Japanese-American men. Men who didn't drink coffee were five times more likely to develop Parkinson's disease than men who drank more than 28 ounces (3½ cups) of coffee per day.[21]

Heartening News

Although coffee consumption has been blamed for causing or contributing to cardiovascular disease in the past, massive population studies find coffee innocent on this count. The *Journal of the American Medical Association* reports no link between coffee and heart disease as determined through a prospective study involving more than 85,000 women.[22] Another study examining more than 45,000 men also showed no link between coffee containing caffeine and cardiovascular disease.[23] These very large studies strongly suggest there is no real-life relationship between coffee consumption and heart disease.

Coffee's Other Health Benefits

While coffee has no definite effect in either direction on heart disease, it definitely improves asthma symptoms. Two large studies, one performed in the United States[24] and one in Italy,[25] showed a decrease of asthma among people who drink coffee. This is probably because caffeine is similar in its chemical structure to theophylline, an effective prescription asthma medication.

If you suffer from occasional headaches, coffee may help. One of the active ingredients in Excedrin, the popular headache medicine, is caffeine equivalent to the amount found in about 1½ cups of coffee. Coffee can stop certain types of headaches, particularly migraine headaches, in their tracks.

Studies show coffee drinkers are significantly less likely to develop gallstones and kidney stones when compared with non–coffee drinkers. After adjusting for variables, one large study from the Brigham and Women's Hospital showed each cup of coffee consumed per day resulted in a 10 percent decreased chance of developing kidney stones in women.[26] A ten-year prospective study following 46,008 men found that men who consistently drank two to three cups of regular coffee daily had a 40 percent decreased risk of symptomatic gallstone disease as compared with men who did not drink coffee.[27]

You Can Have Your Latte, but Hold the Sugar and Fat

You certainly don't have to drink coffee on the Gold Coast Cure. However, by now you should be convinced coffee is not a vice after all. You may drink coffee as long as you do not add sugar to it. Splenda brand sweetener or stevia are good alternatives. You can use low-fat, all-natural dairy products and even light cream to flavor your coffee so long as you keep track of the total amount of saturated fat you consume. Remember, no more than 15 to 20 grams of saturated fat per day is allowed. Cream substitutes and "whiteners" containing hydrogenated oils, partially hydrogenated oils and omega-6 vegetable oils are forbidden. It goes without saying you positively *must* steer clear of those sugar-sweetened coffee-like beverages at doughnut shops and coffeehouses.

BOTTOM LINE ───────────────────────────────────────

Coffee is acceptable on the Gold Coast Cure.

Tea Time

The health benefits associated with drinking tea have been touted for centuries. In addition to the caffeine in tea, it offers its own unique set of impressive antiaging antioxidants. A growing body of scientific evidence links tea drinking with better health and a decreased risk of developing several chronic diseases.

All three types of caffeinated tea (green, black and oolong) contain powerful antioxidants called flavonoids (also known as tea polyphenols), special phytochemicals shown to be helpful in fighting inflammation and infection. The flavonoids in tea have strong antioxidant capabilities. For example, tea flavonoids have been shown to inhibit oxidation of "bad" LDL cholesterol,[28] which could decrease your tendency to develop artery disease.

Regular tea drinkers who had one or more cups of tea per day were recently shown to have a 44 percent decreased risk of suffering from a heart attack as compared with those who didn't drink tea.[29] In another study in which almost five thousand people were followed for an average of five and a half years, tea drinkers were shown to have a markedly decreased risk of having a heart attack or dying from a heart attack as compared with people who did not drink tea.[30]

The Third International Scientific Symposium on Tea and Human Health (yes, such an event exists!) held in 2002 presented research supporting tea's potential to promote health and reduce the incidence of chronic disease. An epidemiological study conducted in Russia was presented showing women who consumed high levels of tea had a 60 percent reduction in their risk of developing rectal cancer as compared with women who drank smaller amounts of tea.[31] Some researchers believe the flavonoids in tea interfere with one or more of the cell-damaging processes that ultimately lead to cancer.

Black or Green?

The primary difference between black and green tea is that green tea is dried out before it has a chance to ferment whereas black tea is allowed to ferment before it is dried. Green tea typically contains more antioxidants than black tea because the fermentation process can destroy some of tea's antioxidants. If you really want to get the absolute most out of tea, it's probably better to choose green tea.

Green tea has been associated with a decreased risk of breast, pancreatic, colon, esophageal and lung cancers in human studies. In one large California study, green tea—but not black tea—was associated with a nearly 50 percent reduction in the risk of developing breast cancer.[32]

Herbalists use green tea to help prevent bacterial infections, reduce tooth decay, lower blood sugar levels and reduce the inflammation associated with arthritis. We are also aware of recent claims that green tea can help with weight loss. In the December 1999 issue of the *American Journal of Clinical Nutrition,* researchers studied the effects of green tea extract on ten young, healthy men. They concluded that green tea has thermogenic properties that promote fat oxidation beyond what could be explained by the tea's caffeine content.[33] Although we are not promising anything, green tea may help you work toward achieving a lower body fat percentage.

The Last Word

While we prefer green tea, we are certainly not against drinking black tea. Both beverages contain natural plant antioxidants called polyphenols that can protect against chronic disease. Don't forget about herbal tea, either. In general, herbal teas have not been studied quite as carefully as standard teas. There are far too many types of herbal tea out there for us to make specific recommendations. However, black tea, green tea and herbal tea alike are perfectly acceptable and encouraged as part of our Gold Coast Cure.

The same rules that go for coffee apply to tea. Don't add sugar. You may flavor tea with Splenda or stevia or with low-fat milk or soy milk. There's no upper limit on tea consumption. And, as is the case with alcohol and coffee, you do *not* have to drink tea on our Gold Coast Cure if you prefer not to.

BOTTOM LINE —————————————————————————————
You can drink all the tea you want on the Gold Coast Cure.

Now that you know what beverages are allowed, it's time to do a complete Kitchen Shape-Up.

Part Three

The Gold Coast Diet and Lifestyle Plan

The Kitchen Shape-Up: Giving Your Pantry a Gold Coast Makeover

Now it's time to put what you've learned into practice. Creating a well-stocked kitchen is critical to making the Gold Coast Cure lifestyle work for you.

To whip your kitchen into shape you must apply the same rules you'd use when reorganizing your clothes closet. The first step in any closet revamp is to toss out or give away the clothes you no longer wear. Likewise, it's time to toss the foods you and your family will no longer eat. Before you can begin to fill your refrigerator and pantry with healthful whole foods, you've first got to free up some space. Aside from freeing up room, tossing the junk removes the temptation to eat those foods you now know are bad for your health and your waistline. Then you'll be able to fill your cabinets with delicious, nutrient-rich food that will give you energy and keep you looking and feeling terrific.

Getting Rid of the Junk: The Toss-It Checklist

Some of you may object to the concept of throwing out "perfectly good" food. We're not asking you to do this: We're only asking that you throw out junk food that has been proven to harm the health of you and your loved ones.

Don't get nervous as you read the "toss-it/save-it" checklist. There are plenty of all-natural, better-tasting alternatives to every single one of the processed foods you'll be tossing, and you may find out that some of your favorite foods are allowed on the Cure.

1) **Toss:** All of the following unhealthful carbohydrate foods that contain enriched flour, wheat flour, unbleached flour or bleached flour as either of their first *two* ingredients.

   You will need to inspect all of the following pantry foods with an eagle's eye:

   - bagels
   - biscuits
   - boxed mixes for preparing cookies or cakes
   - breads
   - bread crumbs
   - breakfast bars
   - breakfast cereals (*dry or hot*)
   - cakes
   - cookies
   - crackers
   - flour
   - muffins
   - pancakes
   - pizza crusts
   - corn chips or "crisps"
   - rolls
   - pretzels
   - waffles
   - most "diet" versions of any of the above foods

NOTE: *You may save once-per-day "sweet" treats. These treats may contain enriched flour as long as they are all-natural and are not made with either hydrogenated oils or partially hydrogenated oils. Put these treats in the back of your pantry so you won't be tempted by them if you're not hungry. (See page 120.)*

Save: Foods that contain whole wheat, any other whole grain, whole-wheat flour, or any other whole-grain flour such as whole-rye flour as the first or second ingredient. If it's still not clear whether or not to toss, then look at the total fiber content and the total carbohydrate content. *If there are not at least 2 grams of fiber per 25 grams of carbohydrate, then the food in question should be tossed.*

2) **Toss:** All white pasta.

   Save: Whole-wheat or whole-grain pasta.

3) **Toss:** All white and all instant rice.

   Save: Brown rice and wild rice.

4) **Toss:** All vegetable shortening and all standard margarines. Standard margarines are margarines that contain either partially hydrogenated oils, hydrogenated oils or both.

   Save: Butter and Earth Balance or Smart Balance spreads.

5) **Toss:** Any and all foods made with hydrogenated oils or partially hydrogenated oils. Carefully read labels on the following foods to determine if they contain these unhealthful oils. Any amount is too much! Read the ingredients list. Trans fats may be present in:

   - biscuit and bread mixes
   - breads and baked goods
   - cake mixes
   - canned sauces
   - cereals
   - cocoa mix
   - cookies
     (even Fig Newtons!)
   - ice cream
   - fish sticks
   - frosting
   - frozen meals and miscellaneous frozen foods
   - granola bars, snack bars, "diet" bars and "energy" bars
   - miscellaneous snack foods

- peanut butter
  (*all-natural nut butters
  should not be tossed*)
- frozen desserts
- potato chips, "crisps" or
  corn chips you missed
  earlier

- microwave popcorn
- soups and soup cups
- waffles

Save: All-natural foods made with healthful, nondamaged fats such as extra-virgin olive oil, canola oil or butter.

6) **Toss:** Processed foods containing heat-damaged, refined omega-6 oils. This basically means you need to toss many of the grocery store vegetable oils you normally use for cooking, and you must also toss processed foods containing these oils. Look closely at the salad dressings you use; most commercial brands contain highly processed vegetable oils. There is no reason to eat these oils. You can get all the omega-6 essential fat you need by eating a well-balanced Gold Coast Cure diet that includes healthful omega-6 whole foods such as nuts, grains and seeds. Refined omega-6 oils are empty calories just like sugar and enriched flour. Furthermore, these oils worsen many types of inflammation when they are eaten in excess. Toss the following vegetable oils and toss any canned, boxed or refrigerated products containing these oils:

- corn oil
- cottonseed oil
- peanut oil
- "pure" vegetable oil

- sesame seed oil
- standard safflower oil
- standard sunflower oil
- soybean oil

NOTE: *Vegetable oils are often hidden in processed vegetarian foods such as soy burgers and veggie burgers, so read labels carefully. There is no reason to pay extra money for soy burgers that contain 50 percent unhealthful processed omega-6 fat. DO NOT GO OVERBOARD. Some vegetable oils should be saved.*

Save: High-oleic sunflower oil, high-oleic canola oil, high-oleic safflower oil and, especially, extra-virgin olive oil—these are all great for cooking and are perfectly safe ingredients in packaged foods. High-quality "expeller-pressed" canola oil is good for homemade no-heat recipes and is also an acceptable ingredient in packaged foods. Quality walnut oil and avocado oil purchased at health food stores are fine. Don't throw out the flax oil either!

7) **Toss:** All processed foods containing "sugar" as the first or second ingredient. You need to scan the ingredient list of many packaged foods carefully because food manufacturers love to disguise sugar by using a variety of misleading terms. Added sugars often appear on food labels as brown sugar, corn sweetener, corn syrup, dextrose, fructose, fruit juice concentrate, glucose, high-fructose corn sweetener, honey, cane juice, malt syrup, maltose, molasses, raw sugar or sucrose.

Save: Most sweet condiments. While sweet condiments such as jelly, catsup, barbecue sauce and others often contain sugar, these products are acceptable *if they are used in moderation* as condiments to flavor otherwise healthful meals and snacks. Moderation for condiments means roughly a tablespoon.

Your Daily Sweet Treat

You can still enjoy one small "sweet treat" each day. As a general rule of thumb, rich desserts such as cheesecake, crème brûlée, brownie, pie or cake should be no larger than about 1 inch thick and half the size of your palm. Servings of ice cream, puddings, mousse and soufflé should be no larger than a half cup. Lighter desserts made with fruit and flour only, containing a minimal amount of fat or cream, such as apple crisp, can be about 1 inch thick and the size of your entire palm but no more!

Your "sweet treat" positively must be all-natural and must not contain hydrogenated or partially hydrogenated oils. Also, please do not treat packaged products containing added sugar as health foods. For example, if you choose to eat a sweet granola bar or a sugar-sweetened packaged cereal, you must treat this product as your "dessert." That means no homemade cheesecake and no all-natural ice cream after dinner. Carefully read labels on all the processed foods you eat, including "granola" bars and "health" bars. If you love the taste of sweets all through the day, try foods made with the Splenda brand sugar substitute instead.

BOTTOM LINE ⎯⎯⎯⎯⎯⎯⎯⎯⎯⎯⎯⎯⎯⎯⎯⎯⎯⎯⎯⎯⎯⎯⎯⎯

Toss anything containing sugar as its first or second ingredient unless you intend for that food to be your one sweet treat allowed each day or unless you can honestly describe that food as a condiment.

8) **Toss:** Sugary drinks. This includes soda and sugar-sweetened fruit drinks. If you are overweight you should strongly consider tossing pure fruit juices too. Unless you're extremely active and you really need the extra calories, it's best to eat whole fruit instead.
   Save: Whole fruits and, only if extremely active, 100 percent fruit juice without added sugar.

9) **Toss:** Fake cheese products, "fat-free" cheese products and all processed cheese foods.
   Save: All-natural, gourmet, full-fat cheeses; all-natural low-fat cheeses; and all-natural "light" cheeses as long as they are *not* "fat free" artificial foods. Soy cheese is also healthful and should not be tossed. Whipped cream cheese is acceptable.

10) **Toss:** Fatty cold cuts such as bologna and salami, bacon, beef sausages, pork sausages, and hot dogs.
   Save: Chicken- and turkey-based cold cuts as well as turkey burgers or turkey sausage as long as you count the saturated fat content toward your daily limit and as long as they are made from all-natural ingredients.

11) **Toss:** Prebreaded meats and fish (chicken nuggets and fish sticks). These products contain refined flour and unhealthful oils.

   Save: Most likely nothing in this category can be saved, unless they have been prebreaded with 100 percent whole grains and were made using extra-virgin olive oil.

That should just about do it! Your cupboard might seem bare by now, but your efforts will be rewarded. There's plenty of great-tasting whole foods in store for you.

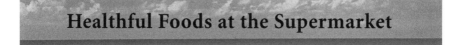

Healthful Foods at the Supermarket

The secret to creating great-tasting healthy meals on short order is planning ahead, because it's a lot easier to tap into your creative side if the necessary ingredients are at your fingertips. Going to the grocery store once a week is crucial to having healthful, fresh ingredients on hand at all times.

While grocery shopping is not everybody's idea of fun, with a little organization, your weekly shopping trips can be less of a hassle. Start by creating a standard master list of all of the basic foods you need to have on hand. Instead of haphazardly writing down food items all over the place, organize the foods you buy into categories. Healthful food categories include fruits, vegetables, meats, fish, dairy, spices and condiments, canned goods, whole-grain breads, and so on. Keep your master list in a convenient location in the kitchen (or on your computer, so it can be printed out as needed), then add foods to your list as supplies run low. Organizing food items by category streamlines your shopping trip and saves precious time.

Planning meals ahead of time is another way to ensure healthful eating—and with a shopping list that takes into account what you'll actually be using, you'll be unlikely to buy more or less food than you need. It should only be necessary to shop about once a week. Try planning one week's worth of meals the day before you shop. Estimate how many breakfasts, lunches and dinners you and your family will eat at home and how many times you'll eat out. After deciding how many times you'll be eating at home, jot down the recipes you intend to make, then write the ingredients for each recipe on your master list under each food category. The entire process takes no more than fifteen minutes—and makes enjoying healthful meals a snap. If you're too busy to cook every night, but love eating home-cooked meals, we suggest you cook only three or four nights a week. What about the other nights? Leftovers! Make use of your freezer too. Many whole foods recipes can be made in bulk and frozen. Casseroles, chili and even meat dishes can be kept frozen or refrigerated for quite some time. It takes about as much work to prepare one recipe for twelve servings as it does preparing one recipe for four servings, so try doubling or tripling your recipes and serving leftovers. (Family members who complain are welcome to cook something else instead.)

Keep in mind that you'll probably need to visit your local natural foods store on occasion to purchase specialty health items such as flax oil, flaxseeds and healthful alternatives to some of your favorite packaged foods. Some urban and suburban grocery stores do stock these items, and full-size health foods supermarkets are growing in number. Nevertheless, in many parts of the country you'll need to make a second stop. The Internet is also a great resource for many specialty food items.

Let the Spree Begin

We'll start with the supermarket, where the vast majority of the foods you need to purchase are readily available. Because most grocery stores are arranged by food category and you've organized your list using these same categories, with just a little practice you'll be able to fly through the store, buying only healthful whole foods.

Vegetables

Eat at least two large servings of vegetables every day. A serving is roughly the size of your closed fist. Aim to eat at least one vegetable with lunch and one with dinner. Most people don't have time to cook vegetables for lunch, so take advantage of precut raw vegetables such as carrots and prepackaged salads. For dinner, choose either fresh or frozen vegetables. Try to eat a wide variety in order to obtain as wide an assortment of micronutrients as possible. The broader the range of colors you incorporate into your diet, the better.

Fruit

All fruits are healthful whether they are fresh, frozen or dried. Look for dried fruit that doesn't contain added sugar or added oil. Avoid fruits canned in sugary syrups.

Other Essential Produce

These foods are sold alongside the fruits and vegetables and should definitely be near the top of your grocery list:

- **Avocado.**
- **Dense Carbohydrates**. Don't forget corn, potatoes and sweet potatoes.
- **Fresh Herbs.** Herbs contain important micronutrients in a delicious, calorie-free package. Many of our recipes call for fresh herbs. To obtain the best possible flavor, try not to substitute dried herbs when the recipe calls for fresh.

- **Garlic.**
- **Olives.**
- **Tofu.** Most supermarkets stock tofu in the fresh produce department. Purchase extra firm tofu to use as an entrée for grilling,
  baking and sautéing and soft or silken tofu for use in custards,
  miso soup, salad dressing, shakes and desserts.

Ingredients for Fresh Salads

Salads are one of the easiest, most convenient ways to meet your
lunchtime vegetable quota. If you choose healthful ingredients and
bulk your salad up sufficiently, you've got a quick, delicious, nutritious, complete lunch. Start with salad greens, the darker the better,
then add your favorite raw vegetables. Save time by purchasing prechopped raw vegetables. Next, add the following salad toppers to create a complete, satisfying meal:

- **Dense Carbs.** Beans, boiled and sliced potatoes (keep the skin
  on!), corn and even whole-grain croutons are all great choices.
  You can make your own healthy croutons at home by cutting
  whole-grain bread into cubes, brushing the bread with extra-
  virgin olive oil and sprinkling with some salt, then baking at 400
  degrees until crispy. Another way to bulk up your salad is to add
  precooked whole grains such as quinoa, wheat berries, whole-
  grain pasta or barley. (You can make these in bulk prior to the
  workweek.)
- **Protein.** Every meal should contain at least some protein. Grilled
  chicken, perhaps left over from last night's dinner, is a good
  choice. Canned chicken, canned tuna, canned sardines and
  canned salmon, packed in water, not vegetable oil, all make convenient, healthful salad toppings. Other ideas include hard-
  boiled eggs, low-fat cheese, soy cheese and baked tofu.
- **Vinaigrette.** We hope you'll try some of the delicious vinaigrette

recipes we've created from flax oil. However, if you're short on time, just mix either extra-virgin olive oil or flax oil with balsamic vinegar and fresh lemon juice. Another option is to purchase a healthful bottled dressing. You'll find a list on page 144.

- **Salad Extras.** To further jazz up your salad, buy olives, avocado, chopped nuts, seeds, roasted red peppers, sun-dried tomatoes, hearts of palm, baby corn or water chestnuts.

Butcher's Market

Meats are perfectly healthy if you look for the absolute leanest cuts available. When it comes to meat, there are no health advantages to selecting fattier cuts. Even if you buy a lean cut of meat, you still need to trim off any remaining visible fat. We're a bit neurotic about visible fat on meat so we use kitchen shears. It's easier to remove excess fat with scissors than with a knife.

- **Chicken:** Consider buying free-range chickens that are raised on healthy, hormone-free diets and are free to forage for most of their food. The result is a thinner, healthier chicken with superior flavor. All chickens store the majority of their fat just under their skin so be sure to avoid eating the skin. Because white meat has less saturated fat than dark meat, it's always the better choice.
- **Beef:** Consider buying hormone-free, grass-fed meats when possible (for more information visit *www.eatwild.com* or *www.americangrassfedbeef.com*). Good cuts of beef include the round tip, top round, eye of round, top loin, tenderloin, filet mignon, sirloin and extra lean ground beef. A serving of beef is about the size of your palm.
- **Pork:** The leanest cuts of pork include the tenderloin, top loin chop, center loin chop and loin roast. Trim all visible fat.
- **Veal:** Tenderloin and the top loin are the leanest cuts of veal.

Keep in mind that veal contains more saturated fat than poultry so it should be an occasional treat, not a staple.

- **Lamb:** Lamb contains more folate and more omega-3 fat than any other red meat. Be sure to trim off any and all visible fat before cooking.

- **Turkey:** Just like chicken, white meat turkey has much less saturated fat than the dark meat. Extra-lean ground turkey is a surprisingly tasty alternative to ground beef. Be cautious of turkey that does not specifically say "extra-lean" because it's possible for ground turkey to contain nearly as much saturated fat as ground beef. Try turkey burgers, turkey meatloaf and even turkey meatballs as more healthful alternatives to beef-based foods.

Fish Market

When buying fish the rules are simple: All unprocessed, unpackaged seafood is good. Prepared, prebreaded, processed products such as fish sticks and crab cakes are almost always a bad choice unless you make them yourself with whole-grain bread crumbs and cook them in healthful, heat-safe oils. Read labels carefully when buying packaged fish.

You must eat three to four servings of fish every week for optimal health—the fattier the fish, the better. If you can't or won't cook fish, you can always buy smoked salmon (lox), smoked trout, or canned salmon, sardines or tuna. Be sure to buy canned fish packed in water or olive oil and avoid canned fish that has been packed in soybean oil or any other vegetable oil. Shellfish is great, too. Shrimp, lobster, crab, oysters, mussels and scallops are all encouraged on the Cure.

- **Frozen Fish:** "Fresh" fish and "frozen" fish taste better than the "fresh from frozen" fish most often available at the grocery store. "Fresh from frozen" fish should be eaten on the day of purchase. If you buy frozen fish, keep it frozen until you're ready to cook it.

The key to fresh-tasting fish is to freeze it only once. Don't allow frozen fish to thaw if you plan to re-freeze it. If you must freeze fish, it's best if it is frozen in water. Just fill a ziplock plastic bag with water, put your fish into the bag, then freeze.

• **Fresh Fish:** To ensure you buy only the freshest-tasting "fresh" fish, try to shop at a market that has a high turnover and preferably one that displays the entire fish. If the entire fish is displayed, look for clear as opposed to cloudy eyes and red gills. Ask the fishmonger which fish is the freshest. (If you just ask whether his fish is fresh, obviously he will respond with a "yes.") Fresh fish should never smell fishy and should always be firm to the touch.

Dairy Case

Now, it's on to the dairy case.

• **Eggs:** Look for omega-3 enriched eggs, the healthiest eggs available. We like Eggland's Best brand because they are 100 percent hormone-free, contain 100 milligrams of omega-3 fat per egg and have 25 percent less saturated fat than regular eggs.

• **Cheese:** Look for all-natural cheeses and consider buying organic when possible. Many supermarkets across the country now carry organic cheese. We especially like Organic Valley and Wholesome Valley Organic cheeses. Purchase regular, "light" or "low-fat" cheese. Save full-fat cheese for gourmet meals on special occasions. Avoid "fat-free" cheese products completely. These foods almost always contain unrecognizable additives and ingredients. "Fat-free" cheeses don't cut it in the taste department, either. If you stick to low-fat or light cheese, we promise you'll barely notice the difference in taste and texture compared with regular cheese. All of the cheeses we list below are easy to find at your local grocery store and all are delicious:

1) **Feta.** "Light" feta cheese gives exceptional flavor to Mediterranean salads.

2) **Low-fat shredded mozzarella.** Rich in calcium, mild in flavor and very versatile.

3) **Low-fat cheese.** The fewer additives the better. Our favorite low-fat cheeses include Laughing Cow Light Gourmet Cheese Bites, Litedammer, King's Choice Light, Havarti, Cracker Barrel 2% Milk Reduced-Fat Sharp White Cheddar, Laura Chenel's Chevre Goat's Milk Cheese and Boursin Light.

4) **Fresh buffalo mozzarella.**

5) **Fresh Parmesan and shredded Parmesan.** A little goes a long way. Very distinctive flavor. Great for gourmet dishes. Low in saturated fat.

6) **Fresh Romano and shredded Romano.** Again, a little goes a long way.

7) **Goat cheese.**

8) **Low-fat cottage cheese** teams well with fresh fruit and, believe it or not, chili.

- **Soy Milk.** We like Sun Soy and Silk brands, which are relatively easy to find. Organic Valley soy milk is also delicious. All contain almost insignificant amounts of added sugar.

- **Rice Milk.** If you're lactose intolerant, you may want to consider buying rice milk.

- **Low-Fat Milk and Skim Milk.** Consider buying organic milk when possible. Organic milk is produced without the use of antibiotics, pesticides and synthetic hormones. Many supermarkets across the country stock organic milk. We especially like Organic Valley low-fat milk. Go to *www.organicvalley.com* for more information. Avoid full-fat milk except for use in special recipes. Whole milk is too high in saturated fat to be recommended for daily drinking.

A Calcium-Rich Treat for Kids

Make a treat for your kids by mixing milk with a little cinnamon and a dash of honey. We created this for our son at a coffee shop one day, and now he always asks for his "special milk treat."

- **Low-Fat Plain Yogurt** is rich in protein and calcium. Avoid brands that contain added sugar unless you intend for that cup of yogurt to be your "sweet treat" for the day. As a general rule of thumb, any low-fat yogurt containing more than about 130 calories per 8 ounces of product contains too much sugar. If you want increased sweetness, add fresh fruit and Splenda brand sugar substitute to plain unsweetened yogurt. We love the Stonyfield Farms organic brand of plain yogurt as a base. Either the "low-fat" version or the "no-fat" version is fine. We also enjoy kefir, which you will probably have to purchase at the natural foods store. We like 2-percent reduced-fat Helios brand kefir the best. This product is loaded with calcium and vitamins, and even contains fiber.
- **Butter.** Purchase organic butter when possible. Many supermarkets across the country stock organic butter. When it comes to butter, moderation is important. One teaspoon contains 2½ grams of saturated fat, so it should go a long way! Try whipped butter, which contains about half the saturated fat as regular butter but all of the taste and flavor. All-natural Land O' Lakes Soft Baking Butter with Canola Oil contains less saturated fat than butter but tastes and bakes just like butter.

- **Butter Alternatives.** While standard margarines are big fat no-nos, there are all-natural butter alternatives on the market that taste sensational and are free from deadly trans fats. We like Smart Balance, especially Smart Balance Omega Plus, and Earth Balance. At only 2½ grams of saturated fat per tablespoon these products are healthier than butter. Smart Balance Light with Flax Oil contains 300 milligrams of omega-3 fats per serving and only 1.5 grams of saturated fat. Do *not* cook with these spreads because they contain heat-sensitive essential fats. Use them instead as spreads or to top hot vegetables, potatoes, corn and so forth, *after* they are done cooking.
- **Crème Fraiche.** Tablespoon per tablespoon crème fraiche contains half as much saturated fat as butter yet tastes every bit as rich. Crème fraiche is great in sauces and can be blended with Splenda and topped with fresh fruit for a simple dessert.
- **Whipped Cream Cheese.** You get all the great taste and smooth texture of real cream cheese with half the saturated fat. One tablespoon provides about 40 calories and only 2½ grams of saturated fat.

Nuts, Seeds and Nut Butters

- **Nut Butters.** Always purchase all-natural nut butters that contain no sugar and no hydrogenated oils or partially hydrogenated oils. You'll find the widest selection at the natural foods store or in the health-foods section of your supermarket. Try all-natural peanut butter, cashew butter and almond butter.
- **Dry-Roasted Soybeans.** These are great for snacking, but be sure they are not roasted in oil.
- **Nuts and Seeds.** Avoid nuts and seeds that have been roasted in oil. Purchase only nuts that are either dry roasted or "raw." Look for peanuts, walnuts, macadamia nuts, cashews, almonds,

hazelnuts, pecans, sesame seeds, pistachios, sunflower seeds, pumpkin seeds and so forth. All varieties of nuts and all varieties of seeds are good for you.

• **Tahini.** This Mideastern spread is made from ground sesame seeds and is rich in essential fat with a strong, distinctive flavor. It's a healthful, tasty alternative to butter and margarine when used to top whole-grain bread. We use it as an ingredient in our homemade vegetable dips, hummus and salad dressings.

Oils, Salad Dressings, Sauces and Condiments

• **Oils.** Do not buy any oils, except for extra-virgin olive oil, at the grocery store. Instead, check out the higher-quality products sold at natural foods stores.

  • **For No-Heat Recipes:**

  Best Choice: Flax oil. You'll have to purchase this oil at the natural foods store.

  Second-Best Choice: Extra-virgin olive oil. May be purchased at any supermarket.

  Third-Best Choice: High-quality, expeller-pressed canola oil. It's best to purchase this product at the health foods store to ensure it is indeed higher quality. Expeller-pressed walnut oil is also acceptable.

  • **For Cooking:**

  Best Choice: Extra-virgin olive oil.

  Second-Best Choice: Extra-virgin coconut oil. Sold at higher-quality supermarkets and at the natural foods store. Butter is also safe.

  Third-Best Choice: High-oleic canola oil, high-oleic sunflower oil or high-oleic safflower oil. Great when a mild flavor is necessary. Sold at higher-quality supermarkets and most natural foods stores. If you can't find these products ask for assistance. They are readily available.

• **Tomato Sauce.** To make healthful, gourmet cooking easy, you should definitely find a tomato-based sauce you love. Almost everyone (even finicky kids) loves tomato sauce! Rich in nutrients, including the antioxidant lycopene, all-natural tomato sauce counts as a "vegetable" serving. Store-bought tomato sauce is great, especially when you've suffered through a busy work day and are too tired to cook. When looking for tomato sauce, follow these three guidelines to ensure you choose the healthiest, best-tasting sauce possible:

1) Avoid sauces that include meat in their ingredient list because they almost always contain too much saturated fat.

2) Avoid sauces made with any type of oil other than extra-virgin olive oil.

3) Avoid sauces that contain any "unrecognizable" ingredients. You want an "all-natural" sauce. These are always the healthiest, best-tasting sauces.

Our favorite brands include, in no particular order:

Rao's Homemade Marinara. Fabulous! Rao's sauces originated in a New York restaurant and the quality is truly unsurpassed in a bottled sauce. The only downside is the price tag.

Gia Russa. These sauces have a homemade quality and richness very similar to the sauces produced by Rao's, but at about half the price.

Victoria Marinara. Scrumptious and reasonably priced, Victoria also makes an amazingly luscious, rich-tasting vodka sauce that is actually low in saturated fat.

Joey Pots and Pans. Made with imported tomatoes, the marinara sauce is absolutely fabulous.

Amy's. All-natural and organic, Amy's offers a wide variety of great-tasting, affordable tomato sauces. Four of our all-time favorite Amy's sauces are Wild Mushroom Pasta Sauce, Puttanesca Pasta Sauce, Garlic Mushroom Pasta Sauce and Tomato Basil Pasta Sauce. You may need to go to the natural foods store to find Amy's brand pasta sauces.

- **Pesto.** A little pesto goes a long way. For the best pesto, select it from the refrigerated section of your supermarket. Be sure it's made exclusively from all-natural ingredients and healthful oils—extra-virgin olive oil is best. If your favorite brand of pesto sauce contains too much full-fat cheese, dilute it with fresh basil and added extra-virgin olive oil.
- **Guacamole.** Buy guacamole from the refrigerated section and look for freshness and "all-natural" ingredients. Try the deli counter, or make your own with a little help from the recipe chapter.
- **Salsa.** Salsa can be another trouble-free, tasty way to meet your vegetable quota. As always, look for all-natural ingredients. Browse the deli section of your favorite supermarket. Salsas come in many varieties, so experiment with exotic varieties such as peach-mango or cilantro-lime. We like Amy's all-natural organic salsas such as Black Bean and Corn.
- **Mustard.** No fat, lots of flavor.
- **Vinegars.** Seek out unusual vinegars such as raspberry, champagne, herbed and so forth.
- **Dried Herbs.** Flavor with a health boost.
- **Fish Rubs.** Two or our favorites are Bobby Flay's Red Chili Rub for Fish and Emeril's Fish Rub.
- **Jelly and Preserves.** Look for all-natural jellies and preserves made with only fruit, fruit pectin and sugar. One brand we especially love is St. Dalfour. Jelly is a condiment, so go easy!

- **Gravy.** Pacific Foods All Natural Turkey Gravy and All Natural Beef Gravy are delicious and low in saturated fat.
- **Honey.** Another condiment to be used sparingly.
- **Brown Sugar.** Go easy; use brown sugar as a condiment only.

Sugar Substitute

Splenda is a calorie-free sugar substitute made from sugar that truly tastes like the real thing. You can use Splenda for cooking and baking the same way you would use sugar, though we tend use about half the volume or purchase Splenda Sugar Blend for Baking. You can also use the naturally sweet herb stevia (you will probably need to go to the natural foods store to locate it).

Cereals and Crackers

Most commercial cereals and most grocery store crackers are not good for you. Make sure the cereals and the crackers you choose don't contain hydrogenated or partially hydrogenated oil, bad vegetable oils or excessive sugar. *Cereals and crackers must always contain at least 2 to 3 grams of fiber per 25 grams of carbohydrate. The best dry cereals usually contain 5 or more grams of fiber per 25 grams of carbohydrate.*

You should be able to locate at least some of the healthful cereals and crackers at your local supermarket, but you may also want to check out the natural foods store shopping guide for a wider selection.

- **Old-Fashioned Oats.** Do not use refined "instant" oatmeal. Old-fashioned oatmeal cooks in about two minutes in your microwave. That's "instant" enough in our book!
- **Hodgson Mill Brand Hot Cereals.** Cracked Wheat, Bulgur Wheat with Soy, and Multi Grain with Milled Flaxseed & Soy.
- **Wheat Bran.** As a "fiber booster" add 1 tablespoon to your hot cereal. Each tablespoon contains 2 grams of fiber.
- **Oat Bran.** Delicious as a hot cereal and perfect as a fiber booster

to add to baked goods such as breads and muffins.

- **Wheat Germ.** Add wheat germ to your favorite hot cereal, breads, muffins and even cake. Sprinkle wheat germ onto yogurt or kefir then top with fruit. Kids love its taste and crunch.
- **Uncle Sam Cereal, Uncle Sam Cereal with Berries** and **Uncle Sam Instant Cereal.** These whole-grain cereals contain omega-3 rich flaxseeds and are exceptionally rich in fiber. Uncle Sam cereals are great served warm or cold. Try boosting the nutritional value and fiber content of your baked goods by including Uncle Sam cereal in muffins and even oatmeal cookies. Also try these varieties:
  - Erewhon Organic Instant Oatmeal with added Oat Bran
  - Erewhon Organic Instant Oatmeal Maple Spice
  - Erewhon Organic Instant Oatmeal Apple Cinnamon
  - Erewhon Organic Instant Oatmeal with Raisins, Dates and Walnuts
  - Erewhon Whole Grain Wheat Flakes
  - Erewhon Fruit-n-Wheat
  - Erewhon Kamut Flakes
  - Erewhon Raisin Bran
  - Erewhon Oatbran with Toasted Wheat Germ
- **Alpen "Naturally Delicious Swiss Style Cereal."** Purchase the "no sugar added" version as opposed to the "original" version. Try sprinkling ground flaxseeds on top.
- **Post Shredded Wheat 'n Bran.** Original Post Shredded Wheat and Shredded Wheat Spoon Size are good, too.
- **Raisin Bran.** Most raisin bran cereals are good. No-sugar-added versions are ideal, but even standard Kellogg's Raisin Bran meets Gold Coast criteria.
- **Kashi Heart to Heart Cereal.** This tastes somewhat like Cheerios but better, and it contains more fiber.
- **Kashi GOLEAN Cereal.** Rich in soy protein.
- **Kashi Seven in the Morning Cereal.**

- **Weetabix.** These wheat biscuits are high in fiber and make a quick breakfast.
- **Wasa and Ryvita** brand crackers are two of our favorite brands. Both companies offer a wide selection of hearty, healthful cracker flavors. Spread these crackers with all-natural nut butter and a bit of honey or raisins to create a tasty balanced snack. Another snack idea is to top them with finely chopped olives, all-natural guacamole or hummus.

Deli Dos and Don'ts

Grocery store delicatessens offer plenty of healthful prepared foods. Avoid mayonnaise-based salads and instead opt for vegetable or bean salads made with extra-virgin olive oil. If you like mayonnaise-based salads, you can make your own at home using canola oil mayo. Salsas are another healthy option. We steer clear of deli pasta salads because we've not yet found a deli offering whole-wheat pasta. You can purchase lean cold cuts from the supermarket deli: look for turkey, chicken, lean ham and even lean roast beef as long as you later trim away the fat. Olives and cheese are also acceptable. Opt for low-fat cheese unless it's a special occasion. Many delis sell healthful bean-based soups, but steer clear of the creamy soups unless you know exactly how they were made. Other generally safe deli soups include Manhattan-style chowders, lentil soups, bean soups, vegetarian chili and split pea soup. Pasta soups and soups containing lots of noodles are not good choices.

If your supermarket of choice carries Hannah brand food products (check out *www.hannahfoods.net*), you're in luck. Look for these delicious, healthful spreads in the deli section:

- Hannah Taboule. A very flavorful Middle Eastern spread.
- Hannah Olive Spread.

- Hannah Pico de Gallo. A fresh Mexican salsa.
- Hannah Hommus. Available in many varieties.

Grains, Pasta, Dried Beans, Pancake Mixes, Breads and Flours

- **Dried Beans.** Although dried beans are not as convenient as canned beans, they're a cinch to make. Cooking beans is about as basic as cooking pasta—in other words, it's pretty difficult to mess up. For perfect beans every time, follow our basic bean prep guidelines in chapter 16. Our personal favorites:

Black beans	Mexican beans
Black-eyed peas	Pinto beans
Cannelloni beans	Red kidney beans
Garbanzo beans	Green split peas
Great Northern beans	Yellow split peas
Lentils	

- **Canned Beans.** Canned beans are one of the most healthful convenience foods—loaded with vitamins, minerals, antioxidants and fiber. Eat them alone, make homemade bean dips, or try adding canned beans to soups, chili, whole-grain pasta dishes and salads. To avoid the "canned" flavor, rinse your beans under water and drain before serving.
- **Pasta.** Avoid plain white pasta and buy whole-grain pasta instead. Make sure the word "whole" is in the list of ingredients. We especially love Hodgson Mill brand whole-grain pasta products, some of which are made with both wheat and milled flaxseeds. You may have to go the natural foods store to find an adequate selection of whole-grain pasta, though more and more supermarkets are coming around. If you decide to eat pasta as your entrée, always think "balance." Round out your meal with some vegetables or tomato sauce made with extra-virgin olive oil

and a bit of protein such as turkey meatballs or cheese.

- **Brown Rice.** Avoid the "quick cook" processed varieties, and never buy empty-calorie white rice.
- **Wild Rice.** Wild rice is great by itself, or try mixing wild rice with brown rice.
- **Pilaf Mixes.** For a quick and tasty side dish, look for 100 percent natural Near East brand rice and grain pilaf mixes such as:
  - Rice Pilaf Lentil with 8 grams of fiber per serving
  - Rice Pilaf Toasted Almond with 2 grams of fiber per serving
  - Brown Rice Pilaf Mix with 3 grams of fiber per serving
  - Rice Pilaf Mix Wheat with 9 grams of fiber per serving
  - Roasted Garlic with Brown Rice with 5 grams of fiber per serving
  - Chicken and Herbs with Brown Rice, Barley, and Pearled Wheat with 6 grams of fiber per serving

  NOTE: *For a taste and nutrient boost, add frozen petite peas, chopped nuts and fresh parsley to your pilafs during the last three to four minutes of cooking time.*
- **Tabbouleh.** Time-crunched people may not want to make this wheat dish from scratch, so you can buy Near East Taboule Wheat Salad mix in the grain section of your supermarket. Simply add a fresh tomato, lemon juice and extra-virgin olive oil or flaxseed oil to create an exotic side dish.
- **Barley.** While whole barley contains more nutrients, the "pearled" barley found in most grocery stores is acceptable. Pearled (partially refined) barley contains about 4 grams of fiber per 25 grams of carbohydrate.
- **Couscous.** Purchase only whole-wheat couscous. The Fantastic Foods line of products makes a delicious whole-wheat couscous.
- **Pita Bread.** Whole-grain pita bread is available at most supermarkets. We like the following brands:
  - The Baker Whole Wheat Pita
  - Toufayan Oat Bran Pita
  - Toufayan Whole Wheat Pita

- **Whole-Grain Bread.** You'll probably have to skip your local supermarket's "bread" aisle and go to the "health foods" aisle or the bakery to find healthful bread. Brands we like include:
  - Mestemacher. Try Pumpernickel, Whole Rye Bread, Organic Linseed Bread, 3 Grain Bread and Fitness Bread.
  - Alvarado Street Bakery. Try varieties such as California Style Complete Protein Bread, Sprouted Soy Crunch Bread, Ultimate Kids Bread, Sprouted Wheat Bread and Sprouted Wheat Raisin Bread.

    NOTE: *In some supermarkets Alvarado Street Bakery brand breads are located in the frozen healthful foods section or in the refrigerated foods section near the dairy.*
  - Food for Life Ezekiel 4:9 Sprouted Grain Bread

    NOTE: *In some supermarkets Food for Life brand breads are located in the frozen healthful foods section or in the refrigerated foods section near the dairy.*
  - The Baker. Lots of choices. Try 9-Grain Whole Wheat. The Baker also offers Low Carb Flax bread. While the words "low carb" have no official meaning and low carb does not necessarily mean the food is good for you, this particular low-carb product is all-natural, healthful and rich in fiber.
  - Nature's Own Healthline Sugar Free 100% Whole Grain Wheat. If you love white bread, you should try this healthy alternative.
  - Rudi's Organic Bakery. Honey-Sweet Whole Wheat Bread (*www.rudisbakery.com*). This product holds true to their promise, "Everything good, nothing bad."

A Whole-Grain Chocolate Treat for Kids

If your kids won't eat whole grain bread, try introducing it to them as "chocolate toast." To make this treat, arrange eight all-natural mini chocolate chips such as the Ghirardelli brand on top of a piece of toasted whole-grain bread and pop it in the microwave for a few seconds until the chocolate softens. Spread the chocolate over the toast with a spoon and serve immediately. If your kids like peanut butter, spread a little all-natural peanut butter on the toast before the chocolate. Either way, this after-school snack sure beats cookies.

You should be able to find at least one of these whole-grain breads at your local supermarket. Check the frozen foods section or the natural foods section, or ask customer service to help you locate them. If you can't find any good bread at your supermarket, you'll need to go to your local natural foods store.

- **English Muffins.** Thomas' English Muffins Hearty Grains 100% Whole Wheat. These English muffins do contain a little bit of soybean oil (less than 1 gram per muffin), but if you really love the taste of English muffins these are an acceptable special treat.
- **Whole-Grain Flours.** Look for Bob's Red Mill brand flours:
  - Soy Flour
  - Whole Wheat Flour
  - Dark Rye Flour
  - Whole Grain Spelt Flour
  - Whole Wheat Pastry Flour. Great for making desserts.

Try Hodgson Mill products also. You'll probably need to visit the natural foods store for a wider selection of whole grain flours. Refer to our natural foods store shopping guide on page 155 for a more extensive list. If you don't know what to do with these flours look on the package for recipe suggestions or check out our own recipe collection.

Frozen Foods

- **Frozen Vegetables.** Frozen vegetables are harvested at the peak of freshness and packaged quickly to retain vitamins and minerals. Warm frozen vegetables in your microwave without added water, then either sauté them briefly in extra-virgin olive oil or simply drizzle a bit of extra-virgin olive oil or flax oil on top. We often saute frozen vegetables with fresh garlic or shallots. Frozen vegetables are great for adding into soups, casseroles and tomato sauces.
- **Frozen Fruit.** Frozen fruit is convenient and fantastic in smooth-ies and great in the morning when you'd rather be sleeping instead of chopping.
- **Ice Cream.** All-natural ice cream is a reasonable "sweet treat." If you combine a small scoop (no more than about ½ cup or 4 ounces) of all-natural ice cream with fresh fruit and nuts, the result is right in line with the Gold Coast Cure. Sadly, many ice creams today are made with unhealthful hydrogenated oils and other unrecognizable ingredients that can't possibly be good for you. Ice cream fans must look for all-natural brands. Our favorite, readily available, all-natural ice creams are sold under the Breyers brand name. The ingredients in many Breyers ice creams are as simple and natural as they come; for example, Breyers strawberry ice cream contains only milk, strawberries, sugar and cream. Do watch your portion size: No more than one small scoop. Avoid ice creams containing more than 150 calories per 4 ounces, even if they are all-natural.
- **Frozen Edamame Beans.** These Japanese-style soft soybeans are addictive and good for you. Edamame beans count as a soy serv-ing. Eat them alone or on salads. Kids love them!
- **Veggie Burgers.** Veggie burgers contain fiber and often soy, but

have about one-third the calories of their beef counterparts. However, as always, buyer beware! Not all brands are healthful. Avoid veggie burgers made with hydrogenated oil or unhealthful vegetable oils. Be sure to read the labels. We especially like the veggie burgers offered by the Boca Burger company and by Amy's. For lunch we sometimes broil our veggie burger of choice in the oven, then top it with barbecue sauce and fresh mozzarella cheese. Other great toppings include hummus, roasted red peppers, grilled onions and soy cheese.

> NOTE: *Some veggie burgers are really more of a carbohydrate than a protein. When planning your meal, read the label to see how much protein is in your veggie burger. If your veggie burger contains less than about 12 grams of protein, consider it to be a carbohydrate food and be sure to add some sort of extra protein such as low-fat cheese to create a more balanced meal (such as a glass of milk or a slice of cheese).*

Our favorite veggie burger varieties, and the protein content in each, include:

- Amy's California Burger, 6 grams of protein
- Amy's Texas Burger, 12 grams of protein
- Amy's Chicago Burger, 10 grams of protein
- Amy's All American Burger, 10 grams of protein
- Boca Burger Roasted Onion, 15 grams of protein
- Boca Burger Vegan, 13 grams of protein
- Boca Burger Garden Vegetable, 13 grams of protein
- Boca Burger Grilled Vegetable, 12 grams of protein

Healthier Alternatives to Some Favorite Convenience Foods

If you're lucky enough to have a health-oriented supermarket in your town, you'll have no problem finding the foods we mention in this section. We are huge fans of the Whole Foods Market, the world's largest chain of organic supermarkets. Go to *www.wholefoods.com* to see if there is a store near you. These stores carry a huge variety of name-brand natural food products. If you can't find the brand names we mention in your local supermarket, you can find them at any well-stocked natural foods store.

- **Potato Fries.** It is possible to buy healthful French fries. We especially recommend the Alexia brand of gourmet, all-natural fries. This company offers an extensive selection, including Sweet Potato Julienne Fries, Rissole Potatoes with Garden Herbs, Julienne Fries with Sea Salt, Oven Reds with Olive Oil, Parmesan, and Roasted Garlic, and many more. Make sure the potato fries you purchase are made with only high-oleic oils or olive oil, as opposed to empty-calorie omega-6 vegetable oils.

- **Salad Dressings.** Purchase only dressings made from either extra-virgin olive oil, expeller-pressed canola oil or expeller-pressed walnut oil. We also suggest you make liberal use of our homemade flax oil salad dressing recipes. If you don't have the time or inclination to make your own dressing, your best bet is to look in the natural foods section of your local supermarket or shop for salad dressing at the natural foods store. Some of our favorite store-bought salad dressings are sold under the Annie's Naturals brand name. Always read the ingredients list because not all of Annie's dressings are made with acceptable oils. Many supermarkets carry Annie's Naturals products, but you might want to go to your neighborhood natural foods store to obtain the best possible selection. Ten of our favorite flavors are

  1) Annie's Naturals Balsamic Vinaigrette

  2) Annie's Naturals Organic Buttermilk Dressing

  3) Annie's Naturals Caesar Dressing

  4) Annie's Naturals Cilantro & Lime Vinaigrette

5) Annie's Naturals Cowgirl Ranch Dressing

6) Annie's Naturals French Dressing

7) Annie's Naturals Roasted Red Pepper Vinaigrette

8) Annie's Naturals Organic Thousand Island Dressing

9) Annie's Naturals Tuscany Italian Dressing

10) Annie's Naturals Gardenstyle Dressing

- **Mayonnaise.** Purchase only canola oil–based mayo. If you can't find this product in your local supermarket, you can go to the natural foods store. If you're a big mayo fan, you'll probably like canola oil mayonnaise. With its fresh taste, it has a far better flavor than the standard highly refined vegetable oil you are used to. One of our favorite brands is Spectrum Naturals Canola Oil Mayonnaise.

- **Chips.** Chips are not health food but, as with dessert, we all need a treat now and then. All-natural chips made using good oils do the least damage. Watch your portion size. Read the label to see what a "serving" is, usually about fifteen to twenty chips . . . not half the bag! If you're trying to lose weight, *skip* the chips entirely. Salty snacks are very easy to overeat! Although natural foods stores offer a wide variety of chips, not all of them meet Gold Coast Cure criteria. One brand that often does is Kettle. This company offers healthful, gourmet tortilla chips and potato "crisps" made using expeller-pressed, high-oleic sunflower and safflower oils. As opposed to most "bad" grocery store chips, Kettle products do contain some fiber. The krisps contain more fiber than the chips, so stick with the krisps. Look for the following varieties:
  - Kettle Blue Corn
  - Kettle Sesame Rye with Caraway
  - Kettle Sweet Brown Rice & Black Bean
  - Kettle Five Grain Yellow Corn

- Kettle Little Dippers
- Kettle Sesame Blue Moons
- Kettle Lightly Salted Low Fat Kettle Krisps
- Kettle Hickory Barbecue Low Fat Kettle Krisps
- Kettle French Onion Low Fat Kettle Krisps

Another chip brand we like is Garden of Eatin'. Specifically, we like their black bean tortilla chips, which have an impressive four grams of fiber per serving as well as white rounds tortilla chips with two grams of fiber per serving.

- **Microwave popcorn.**
  - Try Farmer Steve's 100% Organic Popcorn. This healthy and fiber-rich snack contains no trans fat. *www.farmersteve.com.*
  - Newman's Own Organics Light Butter Flavored Pop's Corn or No Butter/No Salt 94% Fat Free Pop's Corn.
- **Whole-Grain Tortilla Wraps.** Food for Life's Ezekiel 4:9 Brand Sprouted Grain Tortillas are delicious.
- **Whole-Grain Pancakes and Waffles.** Some supermarkets and most natural foods stores offer a decent selection of frozen whole-grain pancakes and waffles. If not, you can always make your own from any of the following easy-to-use healthful products:
  - Bob's Red Mill 10 Grain Pancake and Waffle Mix
  - Bob's Red Mill Buckwheat Pancake and Waffle Mix
  - Hodgson Mill Multi Grain Buttermilk Pancake Mix with Milled Flaxseed & Soy
  - Hodgson Mill Buckwheat Pancake Mix
  - Hodgson Mill Whole Wheat Buttermilk Pancake Mix
  - Hodgson Mill Insta-Bake whole-wheat variety baking mix. As the name implies this product is used for more than just pancakes.
- **Frozen Whole-Wheat Waffles.** Look for Vans All-Natural and Organic Waffles (*www.vansintl.com*). You will love the

convenience of these great-tasting and good-for-you waffles:
- Vans Wheat Free
- Vans Wheat Free Flax
- Vans Wheat Free Apple Cinnamon
- Vans Wheat Free Blueberry
- Vans Belgian 7 Grain Waffles

- **Canned Soups and Chili.** Canned soups and vegetarian chili are perfect for lunchtime on the go. Be cautious when purchasing soups and chili because most brands are neither healthful nor the least bit tasty. We've had good luck with Amy's brand soups and chili. Some of our favorite's include:
  - Amy's Medium Chili
  - Amy's Medium Black Bean Chili
  - Amy's Lentil Soup
  - Amy's Split Pea Soup
  - Amy's Lentil Vegetable Soup
  - Amy's Chunky Tomato Bisque

  Another excellent choice would be the gourmet soups made by the Pacific Foods company. Pacific Foods prepared soups come in a "soft" can. We promise their products taste nothing like any canned soup you've ever tried. For starters, try their Creamy Tomato Soup.

- **Baked and Refried Beans.** Try Amy's all-natural and organic baked beans at your next barbecue or the refried beans the next time you make Mexican food.
  - Amy's Vegetarian Baked Beans
  - Amy's Organic Refried Beans with Green Chiles
  - Amy's Refried Black Beans

- **Instant Soups and Instant Chili.** Instant soups are perfect for your on-the-go life. Add hot water, stir and eat! The only problem is in finding brands that are both edible *and* nutritious. Our favorite brand of instant soup is Fantastic Foods. The following varieties all meet Gold Coast nutrition and gourmet taste standards and are all exceptionally rich in fiber. We sometimes add shredded cheese to these soups for extra protein and calcium:

- Fantastic Foods Jumpin' Black Bean
- Fantastic Foods Country Lentil
- Fantastic Foods Split Pea
- Fantastic Foods Cha Cha Chili
- Fantastic Foods Five Bean Soup

- **Energy Bars and Granola Cereal.** Zoe Foods makes a wonderful line of healthy, delicious products containing flax and soy. All Zoe Foods are free from hydrogenated oils and all are loaded with fiber and nutrients. Visit their Web site for more information at *www.zoefoods.com*. These products are especially helpful if you travel a lot. Try the following:

  - Zoe Foods Chocolate Flax & Soy Bar
  - Zoe Foods Apple Crisp Flax & Soy Bar
  - Zoe Foods Peanut Butter Flax & Soy Bar
  - Zoe Foods Lemon Flax & Soy Bar
  - Zoe Foods Cranberries Currants Flax & Soy Granola Cereal
  - Zoe Foods Honey Almond Flax & Soy Granola Cereal
  - Zoe Foods Apple Cinnamon Flax & Soy Granola Cereal

- **Cereal Bars.** Nature's Choice makes great tasting cereal bars from all-natural ingredients, including whole grains such as oats and barley. Try all six delicious flavors:

  - Nature's Choice Multigrain Cherry Cereal Bars
  - Nature's Choice Multigrain Triple Berry Cereal Bars
  - Nature's Choice Multigrain Strawberry Cereal Bars
  - Nature's Choice Multigrain Raspberry Cereal Bars
  - Nature's Choice Multigrain Blueberry Cereal Bars
  - Nature's Choice Multigrain Apple-Cinnamon Cereal Bars

- **Vegetarian Entrees and Meal Helpers.** If you want to eat more tofu but have no idea how to incorporate it into your meals, you will love these Fantastic Foods products. Read the label, follow the directions, add extra tofu and voila! Tasty, soy-based entrees in a flash.
  - Fantastic Foods Nature's Burger
  - Fantastic Foods Sloppy Joe Mix
  - Fantastic Foods Taco Filling
  - Fantastic Foods Tofu Scrambler
  - Fantastic Foods Vegetarian Chili
- **Appetizers and International Foods.** Many modern supermarkets and most natural foods stores offer a wonderful selection of healthful, gourmet ethnic foods. Fantastic Foods manufactures convenient internationally inspired foods. All you need to do is follow the directions on the box. You'll be enjoying a healthful, tasty, internationally inspired appetizer in minutes:
  - Fantastic Foods Falafel (Near East also makes a falafel mix.)
  - Fantastic Foods Instant Black Beans
  - Fantastic Foods Instant Refried Beans
  - Fantastic Foods Spinach Parmesan Hummus
- **Frozen Meatballs.** Look for Nate's brand vegetarian meatless meatballs. They are rich in soy, low in saturated fat, delicious and easy to prepare. Look for the following varieties:
  - Nate's Classic Flavor Meatless Meatballs
  - Nate's Savory Mushroom Meatless Meatballs
  - Nate's Zesty Italian Meatless Meatballs
- **Ostrich Meat.** Look for gourmet and all-natural Blackwing Ostrich meats in the frozen section. As the package says, these ostrich patties really do have all the delicious flavor of beef . . . and yet they are even leaner than chicken! For best results cook medium.
- **Frozen Chicken Nuggets.** Nate's also makes delicious vegetarian "chicken" nuggets. Nate's Chicken Style Nuggets are a tasty,

healthful way to serve soy to finicky children.

- **Frozen Burritos.** Ready-to-eat burritos can be incredibly healthy, nutrient-dense and fiber-rich—if they are made with whole ingredients. For anyone in a hurry, these burritos make a quick, handy lunch. We love Amy's brand frozen burritos. If you can't find these burritos in your supermarket, try the natural foods store.
  - Amy's Bean & Rice Burrito—Non Dairy
  - Amy's Bean & Cheese Burrito
  - Amy's Breakfast Burrito
- **Frozen Entrees.** The next time you are in a hurry for a quick and healthy lunch or dinner try one of the following delicious all-natural and organic meals by Amy's.
  - Amy's Vegetable Lasagna
  - Amy's Tofu Vegetable Lasagna
  - Amy's Black Bean and Vegetable Enchilada
  - Amy's Garden Vegetable Lasagna (Gluten-Free)
  - Amy's Veggie Loaf with Gravy
  - Amy's Indian Samosa Wraps
  - Amy's Indian Palak Paneer
  - Amy's Indian Mattar Paneer
  - Amy's Country Dinner
  - Amy's Chili and Cornbread
- **Frozen Mexican Food.** Mexican food lovers will delight in Nate's wholesome, vegetarian Tacuitos. Look for the following varieties:
  - Nate's Black Bean and Soy Cheese Tacuitos
  - Nate's Chicken Style Tacuitos
  - Nate's Beef Style Tacuitos
- **Cheese Alternative.** Look for Lisanatti Almond cheese. This cheese alternative is actually made from an almond base. It is surprisingly tasty and just like the package claims, it "Shreds, Melts, and Tastes Great!"

- **Prepared Cookies.** If you want an all-natural cookie as your "sweet treat" but don't necessarily want to make your cookie from scratch, a good choice is Country Choice Certified Organic Cookies. They come in a wide variety of flavors sure to please. Some of our favorites include:
  - Country Choice Peanut Butter Cookies
  - Country Choice Double Fudge Brownie Cookies
  - Country Choice Chocolate Chip Cookies
  - Country Choice Oatmeal Raisin Cookies
  - Country Choice Chocolate Chip Walnut Cookies
  - Country Choice Ginger Cookies
- **Whole-Grain Bread Mixes.** Many boxed bread mixes yield the taste of homemade bread without the time and effort. Most natural foods stores provide a good selection of whole-grain bread mixes, though you still need to make sure no enriched flour or refined flour has been added to the mix. Two of our favorite bread mixes are made by Bob's Red Mill:
  - Bob's Red Mill 100% Whole Wheat Bread Mix
  - Bob's Red Mill Cornbread & Cornmeal Muffin Mix
  NOTE: *An easy way to add some fiber and omega-3 essential fat to your diet is to make bread with ground flaxseeds.*
- **Boxed Cake and Cookie Mixes.** Cookies and cake aren't health foods, but they do taste good and you may want to enjoy a little bit now and then as your "sweet treat." As with any "sweet treat" make sure you watch the portion size! Almost all of the boxed cake mixes sold at the supermarket are junk. Purchase only all-natural cake and cookie mixes made without hydrogenated or partially hydrogenated oils. One of our favorite cake mixes is sold by the Dr. Oetker company under the Simple Organics trade name. Arrowhead Mills also makes delicious baking mixes. When making cake at home the only oils you should use are

high-oleic canola oil, high-oleic sunflower oil and high-oleic saf-flower oil. Try the following products:

- Dr. Oetker Simple Organics Chocolate Cake Mix
- Dr. Oetker Simple Organics Marble Cake Mix
- Arrowhead Mills Brownie Mix
- Fearn Banana Cake Mix
- Fearn Spice Cake Mix
- Fearn Carob Cake Mix

For extra fiber, nutrition and taste try adding some oats (any-where from ½ to ¾ of a cup) to the following cookie mixes:

- Arrowhead Mills Oatmeal Raisin Cookie Mix
- Arrowhead Mills Chocolate Chip Cookie Mix
- Arrowhead Mills Peanut Butter Cookie Mix

NOTE: *Avoid ready-made frostings available at the supermarket. They are universally loaded with deadly trans fats and globs of sugar. Homemade frosting is easy to make and tastes delicious. Mix 1 cup (8 ounces) of whipped cream cheese with 3 to 4 tablespoons of powdered sugar, Splenda brand sugar substitute to taste, 2 teaspoons vanilla extract, a gentle squeeze of lemon juice and 2 to 3 tablespoons of light sour cream. If you want to make chocolate frosting, just add unsweetened cocoa, such as Ghirardelli unsweetened cocoa.*

- **Cakelike Sweet Bread.** Sunnyvale Organic and Nature's Path make outstanding, 100 percent healthy cakelike breads containing no added sugar. These breads are rich in fiber and nutrients. They are moist, rich and truly delicious. We're not kidding! Look for the following varieties. For a special treat, try melting a few Ghirardelli chocolates on top of these breads and place in the microwave for ten to fifteen seconds:
  - Sunnyvale Organic Bakery Fruit, Date, and Pecan
  - Sunnyvale Organic Bakery Stem Ginger
  - Sunnyvale Organic Bakery Cherry, Fig, & Orange
  - Sunnyvale Organic Bakery Rich Fruit
  - Sunnyvale Organic Bakery Carrot & Raisin with Almond

- Nature's Path Whole Rye Manna Bread
- Nature's Path Carrot Raisin Manna Bread
- Nature's Path Multi Grain Manna Bread
- Nature's Path Fruit & Nut Manna Bread
- Nature's Path Whole Wheat Manna Bread

- **Whole Grain Cereals.** Whether you like hot or cold cereal, the selection at any natural foods store or any health foods–oriented supermarket is sure to be extensive. Many people do not eat hot cereal because they think it's too time consuming to make. If you have a microwave it should take you no longer than three to four minutes start to finish. To make hot cereal, follow the manufacturer's serving size suggestion. Typically you would use either ¼ cup or ½ cup dry cereal, then add ½ to ¾ cup of soy milk or low-fat milk to the bowl and microwave for a minute or so. Top hot cereal with fresh fruit, nuts, seeds or ground flaxseeds. Hot and cold cereals we like include:
  - Bob's Red Mill Creamy Buckwheat Hot Cereal
  - Bob's Red Mill 10 Grain Hot Cereal
  - Bob's Red Mill 5 Grain Rolled Hot Cereal
  - Bob's Red Mill 7 Grain Hot Cereal
  - Bob's Red Mill 8 Grain Wheatless Hot Cereal
  - Bob's Red Mill Apple, Cinnamon, & Grains Hot Cereal
  - Bob's Red Mill Grains & Nuts Hot Cereal
  - Bob's Red Mill Old Country Style Muesli
  - Bob's Red Mill Spice N' Nice Hot Cereal
  - Hodgson Mill Multi Grain Hot Cereal with Milled Flaxseed & Soy
  - Hodgson Mill Cracked Wheat All Natural Hot Cereal
  - Hodgson Mill Bulgur Wheat with Soy Hot Cereal
  - McCann's Steel Cut Irish Oatmeal
  - Kashi The Breakfast Pilaf, Seven Whole Grains and Sesame

- Nature's Path Organic Flax Plus Multigrain Cereal
- Nature's Path 8 Grain Synergy
- Nature's Path Multigrain Oatbran
- Nature's Path Optimal Slim
- Nature's Path Heritage Bites
- Nature's Path Organic Pumpkin FlaxPlus Granola
- Ezekiel 4:9 Sprouted Grain Cereal: Golden Flax
- Barbara's Bakery GrainShop
- Ezekiel 4:9 Sprouted Grain Cereal: Cinnamon Raisin
- Arrowhead Mills Four Grain Plus Flax Hot Cereal
- Arrowhead Mills Seven Grain Hot Cereal
- Arrowhead Mills Wheat Free Seven Grain Hot Cereal
- Barbara's Bakery Multigrain Shredded Spoonfuls

- **Shortening.** While in general we don't advocate the use of shortening, Spectrum Naturals does offer a product called Organic Shortening that may be used in recipes requiring shortening. The organic palm oil in this product is trans fat–free. This product is lower in saturated fat than butter.

- **Frozen Whole-Wheat Pizza.** The brands listed below are made primarily from whole-wheat flour but do contain a little bit of refined flour. Nevertheless, they contain significantly more fiber than the vast majority of frozen convenience pizzas and much less saturated fat. To boost the fiber and nutritional content even further, add your own fresh vegetables. You will be pleasantly surprised by how tasty the following pizzas are:

    - A.C. LaRocco Cheese and Garlic Pizza (3 g. fiber per serving)
    - A.C. LaRocco Greek Sesame Pizza (3 g. fiber per serving)
    - A.C. LaRocco Garden Vegetarian Pizza (3 g. fiber per serving)
    - A.C. LaRocco Quattro Formaggio Pizza (8 g. fiber per serving)
    - A.C. LaRocco Spinach and Artichoke Pizza (8 g. fiber per serving)
    - A.C. LaRocco Polynesian Pizza (3 g. fiber per serving)

- A.C. LaRocco Tomato and Feta Pizza (3 g. fiber per serving)
- A.C. LaRocco Shitake Mushroom Pizza (3 g. fiber per serving)
- Amy's Spinach Pizza (2 g. fiber per serving)
- Amy's Cheese Pizza (2 g. fiber per serving)
- Amy's Mushroom and Olive Pizza (2 g. fiber per serving)
- Amy's Rice Crust Cheese Pizza (2 g. fiber per serving)
- **Crackers.** Hain Pure Foods Reduced Fat Wheatettes are great-tasting, all-natural crackers children love.

Natural Foods Store Shopping List

We go to the natural foods store about once every other week. What follows is just a partial listing of the healthful foods you can find at the natural foods store. Some of these foods may be new to you, but if you give them a try you won't be disappointed. Unfortunately, many of these products are not yet available at even the most progressive neighborhood supermarkets.

- **All-Natural Nut Butters.** While most any grocery store stocks all-natural peanut butter, the natural foods store will also carry almond butter, cashew butter and often even hazelnut butter. Refrigerate these nut butters after opening.
- **Tahini.** Several brands offering subtle differences in taste will be available. Refrigerate tahini after opening.
- **Canned Soybeans.** Using canned soybeans is a convenient way to incorporate soy into your meals. They have a mild flavor and are quite versatile.
- **Dry-Roasted Soybeans.** Try these as a healthful, delicious fast

food. Be sure to purchase only dry-roasted soybeans and avoid
those roasted in oil.

- **Tempeh.** This Indonesian favorite has a firm texture, a chewy
  consistency and a nutty, mushroom-like flavor. Tempeh is great
  steamed, pan fried, broiled or cooked on the grill. You can sauté
  tempeh in either extra-virgin olive oil or a teaspoon of melted
  butter. Try topping tempeh with cheese or sauce, or serving it
  crumbled into salads, stews and casseroles.
- **Flax Oil.** Our favorite brand of high-quality flax oil is Barlean's.
  Flax oil is rarely in stock at the grocery store. While on the Gold
  Coast Cure you must eat either flax oil or flaxseeds every single
  day. Keep flax oil refrigerated because it's heat sensitive and
  spoils quickly. Do not use flax oil in any recipe requiring heat.
  Purchase only a small amount at any one time, enough to use
  within three to six weeks.
- **Flaxseeds.** High-quality flaxseeds are also offered by Barlean's.
  They call their ground flaxseed product Forti-Flax. You can purchase ground/milled flaxseeds or, alternatively, you can grind
  whole flaxseeds yourself in a coffee grinder. Ground/milled
  flaxseeds should be stored in your freezer once the seal has been
  broken. Unlike flax oil, flaxseeds can be used in cooking. We add
  ground flaxseeds to almost all of the muffins, cakes and breads
  we make. If you don't go overboard, it's impossible to tell the
  difference.
- **Expeller-Pressed Canola Oil.** We like the widely available
  Spectrum Naturals brand. Expeller-pressed canola oil is good for
  no-heat recipes, but it's even better to use flax oil (much more
  omega-3 fat) or extra-virgin olive oil (fewer by-products from
  the refining process) when possible.
- **Cooking Oils.** Purchase only extra-virgin olive oil, high-oleic
  canola oil, high-oleic safflower oil and high-oleic sunflower oil

for cooking. The Spectrum Naturals brand offers a high-oleic canola oil called Super Canola Oil as well as proprietary high-oleic sunflower and safflower oils. Remember, extra-virgin olive oil is always best as this type of oil is minimally damaged by modern mass-production techniques.

- **Gourmet Specialty Oils.** Purchase expeller-pressed avocado oil for use in either no-heat or high-heat recipes. Purchase expeller-pressed walnut oil, which happens to be rich in omega-3 essential fat, for special no-heat recipes. Always purchase these oils from high-quality manufacturers, such as Spectrum Naturals.
- **Stevia.** An all-natural sugar substitute available at most health foods stores.
- **Kefir.** Our all-time favorite is made by Helios. We like the plain 2 percent reduced-fat version. Go to *www.heliosnutrition.com* for more information. Lifeway Low-Fat Plain Kefir is also delicious. Some grocery stores carry kefir.
- **Whole-Wheat Bread Crumbs.** Whole-wheat bread crumbs taste much better than processed white bread crumbs. Natural foods stores carry whole-wheat bread crumbs, or you can make your own. To make homemade bread crumbs, pulse one or two whole-wheat bread slices in a food processor or blender, season with salt, pepper and extra-virgin olive oil, then spread on a cookie sheet and bake in the oven at 350 degrees for five to ten minutes or until lightly browned.
- **Snack Bars.** Look for Save the Forest Organic Trail Mix Bars made by the New England Natural Bakers. Our favorite flavor is Cranberry Crunch. Instead of a cookie, try giving your children one of these more healthful treats; they'll get a healthful dose of nuts and seeds.
- **Crackers with Flax and Seeds.** Dr. Kracker makes delicious, healthful crackers made with flaxseeds and sunflower seeds. Look

for Dr. Kracker Klassic 3 Seed crackers and Pumpkin Seed
Cheese crackers.

- **Whole-Grain Flours.** Both Hodgson Mill and Bob's Red Mill
make a wide variety of nutrient- and fiber-rich whole-grain
flours. You probably haven't heard of most of the flours we list,
but they taste great. Read the package labels. Most flours provide
tasty serving ideas right on the package, or you can visit the
company's Web site for more recipe ideas. Expand your baking
repertoire by discovering the fabulous taste of whole-grain
breads, muffins, cakes and more. Some of our favorites include:
  - Bob's Red Mill Almond Meal Flour
  - Bob's Red Mill 10 Grain Flour
  - Bob's Red Mill Amaranth Flour
  - Bob's Red Mill Barley Flour
  - Bob's Red Mill Black Bean Flour
  - Bob's Red Mill Garbanzo Bean Flour
  - Bob's Red Mill Graham Flour
  - Bob's Red Mill Triticale Flour
  - Bob's Red Mill Pumpernickel Dark Rye Meal
  - Bob's Red Mill Kamut Flour
  - Bob's Red Mill White Bean Flour
  - Bob's Red Mill *or* Hodgson Mill Soy Flour
  - Bob's Red Mill *or* Hodgson Mill Whole Wheat Pastry Flour
  NOTE: *Pastry flour is ground especially for use in "sweet treats."*
  - Hodgson Mill Oat Bran Flour
  - Hodgson Mill Whole Grain Rye Flour
  - Hodgson Mill Organic Spelt Flour
  NOTE: *The Arrowhead Mills company also makes a wide variety of nutritious, organic flours.*
- **Stone-Ground Cornmeal.** Great for making healthful cornbread.
- **Raw Seeds.** As is the case with nuts, seeds must not be roasted in
oil. Purchase sunflower, poppy, sesame and pumpkin seeds.

- **Sauces and Condiments.** At the natural foods store you'll find a wide array of exotic ethnic sauces. Try experimenting with Thai and Indian flavors. If you take advantage of healthful prepared sauces and condiments, you can easily spice up bland-tasting chicken and tofu dishes and add zest to vegetable, bean and whole-grain dishes. Use sauces and condiments at the barbecue, as marinades to flavor fish, poultry and tofu, and as dressings for your whole-grain side dishes. Most sauces and condiments do contain sugar, but the amount you're eating is almost always small. As long as you use condiments as condiments you'll be fine. Be creative. If you lack creativity you can always read the product labeling for suggestions! Some of our favorite sauces and condiments are:
  - Thai Kitchen Thai Barbecue Sauce
  - Thai Kitchen Spicy Thai Chili Sauce
  - Thai Kitchen Lemongrass Splash
  - Thai Kitchen Sweet Red Chili Sauce
  - Thai Kitchen Light Sweet Plum Dipping Sauce
  - Annie's Naturals Original Recipe BBQ Sauce
  - Annie's Naturals Smokey Maple BBQ Sauce
  - Annie's Naturals Organic Honey Mustard
  - Annie's Naturals Organic Horseradish Mustard
  - Annie's Naturals Organic Raspberry Mustard
- **Whole-Grain Spaghetti and Pasta.** A natural foods store will have the widest selection of whole-grain pasta products. We love Hodgson Mill whole-grain pastas, some of which contain ground flaxseeds.
- **Whole-Wheat Pie Shells.** These are great for making quiche and fruit pies but must be made without hydrogenated oil. Look for them in the frozen section of the natural foods store.
- **Pies.** Natural Feast says they make the "healthiest pies in the

world," and they are probably right. These pies are made without hydrogenated oils, and they contain no refined sugar, no additives, no preservatives and no refined vegetable oils. They also contain fewer calories than regular pie. Natural Feast pies are, unfortunately, a bit tricky to locate. You can order online if you wish at *www.NaturalFeast.com*. Our favorite flavors include:

- Natural Feast Apple Gourmet Streusel Pie
- Natural Feast Blueberry Gourmet Streusel Pie
- Natural Feast Chocolate Mousse Pie

- **Whole-Wheat Pizza Crust.** To boost the nutritional content of pizza, buy whole-wheat crust made without hydrogenated oils, and be sure to make your pizza with lots and lots of vegetables. We like to come up with a theme when creating homemade pizza. Some examples:

1) **Italian Perfect Pizza.** Before baking your pizza crust, brush it with a bit of extra-virgin olive oil. Add fresh-sliced tomatoes, drizzle on a bit more extra-virgin olive oil, then add thinly sliced fresh buffalo mozzarella, sliced black olives, fresh basil leaves and crushed garlic.

2) **Greek Goddess Pizza.** Before baking, brush the premade crust with a bit of extra-virgin olive oil, then add lots of fresh spinach leaves, chopped fresh tomatoes, crumbled feta cheese, kalamata olives and pine nuts.

3) **Veggie Lovers Delight.** Cover the pizza crust with your favorite brand of tomato sauce, low-fat mozzarella cheese, frozen corn kernels, sun-dried tomatoes (soaked first in water to rehydrate), sliced red peppers and fresh baby mushrooms. For extra protein, you can always add soy pepperoni slices . . . they sound a bit odd, but they are surprisingly tasty! When your pizza is done, sprinkle white pepper,

salt, oregano and a bit of freshly shaved Parmesan cheese.

4) **South of the Border Pizza.** Cover the pizza crust with your favorite brand of salsa, add drained and rinsed canned black beans, jalapeño peppers or chopped canned green chili peppers, spicy low-fat cheese, and frozen corn kernels. When your pizza is done, top it with fresh-chopped cilantro and low-fat sour cream.

• **Frozen Ravioli.** A ravioli dinner can be healthful. When the "chef" has suffered through a busy, hectic day, ravioli can be a lifesaver. To make a complete meal, find a healthful, all-natural ravioli, add your favorite brand of tomato sauce, sauté a side dish of either fresh or frozen vegetables in extra-virgin olive oil and garlic, then top the whole ensemble with a tablespoon or two of freshly shaved Parmesan cheese. When looking for healthy ravioli, keep in mind the following guidelines:

1) Your ravioli of choice must be made with all-natural ingredients. No hydrogenated or partially hydrogenated oils and no refined vegetable oils.

2) Ravioli should be stuffed primarily with vegetables, not cheese. Avoid ravioli made with meat. These almost always contain too much saturated fat. Packaged ravioli should contain no more than 3 grams of saturated fat per serving.
NOTE: *We admit it's difficult to find ravioli made from whole wheat. We like the Soy Boy brand of vegetarian vegetable-filled ravioli. Although the manufacturer does not use whole-wheat pasta, the other ingredients are all-natural and healthy. This brand of ravioli is low in saturated fat and, because it's filled with vegetables, it's rather rich in fiber despite being made without whole-grain flour. Our favorite variety is Soy Boy Roasted Red Pepper and Tofu Filling with 3.5 grams of fiber, 10 grams of protein and only ½ gram of saturated fat per serving.*

• **Dried Bean Soup Mixes.** The natural foods store usually offers a good variety of dried bean soup mixes made from healthful all-natural ingredients. These soups taste just like homemade and are incredibly easy to make. One of our all-time favorites is Bob's Red Mill 13 Bean Soup Mix.

• **Grains.** Health foods stores offer a wider, more exotic selection of whole grains than the supermarket. Bob's Red Mill sells almost any variety of grain you can imagine, as well as several combination grains. Grains make wonderful, fiber-rich side dishes for either lunch or dinner and are very easily prepared. Make a grain pilaf by sautéing garlic and finely chopped onion in extra-virgin olive oil, then add some chopped nuts, a precooked grain of choice and fresh chopped herbs. Or, simply top your grains with a bit of extra-virgin olive oil or flax oil and a table-spoon of freshly shaved Parmesan cheese. Add grains to soups or salads. Experiment with all of the following whole grains:

- Amaranth
- Buckwheat, also known as kasha
- Whole-wheat couscous
- Millet
- Quinoa
- Whole barley
- Wheat and rye berries
- Bulgur wheat
- Triticale
- Bob's Red Mill 3 Grain Wild Rice Blend
- Bob's Red Mill Wild Rice & Brown Rice

We hope you're convinced: Whole foods living need not be boring. Whole foods really do taste better than processed food, and whole foods are easy to find. Now that your pantry is stocked, it's time to plan your meals in Gold Coast style.

Meal Planning: 2 Weeks of Meals on the Cure

M any health and diet books fail to appreciate the need for "custom-made," client-driven meal planning. Many of these books provide a specific menu everyone is supposed to follow for one, two or even three weeks at a time. The authors suggest that rigid adherence to specific menus is required for weight loss and health maintenance. This doesn't seem reasonable to us, and we think it's a big part of why so many diets fail: they simply don't offer feasible eating plans for real life. Our meal plans are custom-made by you, tailored to your individual taste preferences and your individual energy needs.

Eating Three Balanced Meals a Day

When planning your meals, think nutrition and balance. The earlier sections of this book gave you the lowdown on nutrition. Now it's time to learn how to make balanced meals that will help you lose weight and get healthy.

The most practical way to make the Gold Coast Cure part of your life is to start by eating three balanced meals every day. A balanced meal is composed of:

1) nutrient-rich whole grains (whole-grain pasta, whole-grain bread, brown rice, beans or potatoes)
2) fruits and/or vegetables
3) healthy fat
4) protein

When balanced meals are eaten at regular intervals, your blood sugar level remains stable, your energy level and your mental performance are optimized, and secretion of insulin—the fat-storing hormone—remains low. Your appetite is naturally suppressed and weight loss becomes easier.

Regardless of your activity level and your body weight, eating three balanced nutrient-rich meals each day is the easiest, most enjoyable path toward health, vitality and wellness. Depending on your schedule and your activity level, you may need to eat more or less at mealtimes, and you may also need to eat one or two snacks a day. Healthful snacks are a perfectly acceptable part of our Cure. Never starve yourself! By the same token, snacks are *not* mandatory. It is equally important that you not eat if you're not hungry.

Although some wellness books recommend eating five or six "mini" meals a day, we suggest you stick with the traditional three squares for three important reasons:

1) It's more convenient and more compatible with social and work schedules to eat three relatively large, balanced meals instead of trying to take in five or six "mini" meals every two to three hours. Planning multiple *healthful* "mini" meals is stressful and time-consuming.
2) Eating tiny meals is unsatisfying physiologically and psychologically. Planning healthy "mini" meals requires conscious portion-size restriction at every meal unless you're very active or unless weight gain has never been a problem for you. If you

eat just three meals a day, you can get up from the table feeling full after every meal yet still lose weight, as long as you choose only Gold Coast Cure–approved whole foods.

3) Eating larger meals that provide 20 to 40 percent of your daily calorie needs can increase your metabolism by a few percent or so for the few hours following mealtime. Smaller meals have less effect on your metabolic rate. The faster your metabolism, the faster you will burn calories.

Snacks Are Allowed— And They Don't Need to Be Balanced

Most people, especially people who exercise, find they need to eat at least one snack every day. Many truly active people eat snacks so large they could be considered "mini" meals. This is perfectly fine as long as you eat these snacks only when you're hungry. *Never eat if you're not hungry.*

Snacks should consist only of healthful whole foods, but snacks do not necessarily need to be "balanced." For example, if you're not very active and you get a little hungry between meals, it's perfectly acceptable to eat *just* an apple for a snack. Don't feel you need to add cheese and whole-grain crackers for the sake of "balance" if you're not that hungry. However, if you're rather active and you get hungry for more than just an apple between meals, you should aim for balance. Balanced snacks should consist of a fruit and/or dense carbohydrate, a little bit of fat, and a little bit of protein. The carbohydrates in the fruit and/or dense carbohydrate provide the energy, and fat and protein help ward off hunger.

The Meal Plans

We provide different meal plans based on your gender and activity level. Although we provide meal plans and serving-size suggestions as a convenience to get you started, we don't want you to get hung up on rigid guidelines when following the Gold Coast Cure. In the long run, consistently choosing healthy foods has much more to do with weight loss and health improvement than obsessing over serving sizes and calorie content. The fewer unhealthful foods you eat, the better you'll do in the long run.

Inflexibility regarding portion sizes will inevitably set you up for failure. Instead, learn to listen to your body. Eat only when you're hungry, stop when you're full. Fuel up primarily, ideally exclusively, on healthful, nutrient-rich foods. Limit the portion size of your "sweet treats," not your nutrient-rich meals. If you're following the Cure for weight loss purposes we know this advice is a bit different than what you're used to, but ask yourself if anything you've tried before has really worked.

Until you become more familiar with picking out new healthy whole foods at the supermarket and the natural foods store, we encourage you to make use of our Gold Coast Foods List in planning your meals. The Gold Coast Foods List is broken down into the exact same categories we use in our meal plans. In this list we even provide serving-size suggestions to assist you with your planning.

Use the following guide to determine your activity level. If you only exercise on certain days, or your job duties change considerably from day to day, you may need to adjust your diet on a daily basis. There is nothing wrong with following our "very light" meal plan one day, then following our "moderate" or even our "active" meal plan the next day.

❦ "Very Light" activity involves sitting at a desk the majority of the day, driving a car to work, reading and typing.

❦ ❦ "Light" activity would include shopping, running errands, child care, cooking and light housework. One trip to the grocery store is still very light activity, but several hours spent shopping or running errands bumps you up into the light category.

❦ ❦ ❦ "Moderate" activity includes light daily activity plus a 30- to 35-minute moderate to high-intensity exercise routine such as our Gold Coast Cure workout. Several hours of outdoor work, such as light yard work, would also qualify as moderate activity as long as you are on your feet most of the time.

❦ ❦ ❦ ❦ "Very Active" includes light daily activity plus a 30- to 35-minute moderate to high-intensity Gold Coast Cure workout plus an extra 20 to 25 minutes of aerobic exercise. Alternatively, all day heavy outdoor labor would qualify as very active.

Fast Track to Weight Loss

If you're currently overweight and you follow the meal plans we provide below based upon an honest appraisal of your activity level, you *will* lose weight. The more overweight you are, the faster you'll lose the excess weight. However, if you want to further speed your weight loss, try one or more of the following suggestions. Do *not* skip meals or cheat on our meal plans.

1) Eat only three meals per day. Skip the snacks entirely. Or, try eating a snack one notch below what your current activity level is. For example, if you're currently Very Active, eat a snack based on Moderate activity.

2) Eliminate the daily sweet treat or indulge only in a few small spoonfuls.

3) Do our Gold Coast Cure 30-minute resistance circuit training workout three times a week but add 25 minutes of aerobic exercise to your Gold Coast workout routine once, twice or even three times per week. Do this despite keeping your snack intake at the Light or Moderate activity level.

Women's Basic Meal Plan for Very Light Activity*

Very light activity involves sitting at a desk the majority of the day, driving a car to work, reading and typing.

Breakfast:

❑ 1 serving fruit

❑ 1 serving dense carbs

❑ 1 serving fat *(any type)*

❑ 1 serving protein *(any type)*

❑ coffee or tea *(if desired)*

Lunch & Dinner:

❑ 1 or 2 servings vegetables

❑ 1½ servings dense carbs

❑ 1 serving fat *(any type)*

❑ 1 serving protein *(any type)*

❑ coffee or tea *(if desired)*

❑ 5 ounces of wine is acceptable

   (with lunch or dinner, not both!)

Reminders:

❑ One of your fat servings at some point during the day must be either flaxseeds or flax oil.

❑ One of your protein servings at some point during the day must be either fish or soy.

❑ Limit your saturated fat to 20 grams a day if you are healthy; 15 grams if you have an inflammatory or heart condition. You don't need to count the fat found in fish.

What about the treat?

In addition to your meals and snacks, you are allowed one small sweet treat per day at any time of the day you like. Refer to the Gold Coast Foods List on page 183 to see what our definition of "small" is!

Women's Basic Meal Plan for Light Activity*

🌴🌴

Light activity would include shopping, running errands, child care, cooking and light housework. One trip to the grocery store is still very light activity, but several hours spent shopping or running errands bumps you up into the light category.

Breakfast:

❑ 1 serving fruit
❑ 1 serving dense carbs
❑ 1 serving fat *(any type)*

❑ 1 serving protein *(any type)*
❑ coffee or tea *(if desired)*

Snack:

NOTE: If you don't want to eat a snack, you can incorporate the following food into your breakfast, lunch or dinner instead.
❑ 1 serving fruit

Lunch & Dinner:

❑ 1 or 2 servings vegetables
❑ 1½ servings dense carbs
❑ 1 serving fat *(any type)*
❑ 1 serving protein *(any type)*

❑ coffee or tea *(if desired)*
❑ 5 ounces of wine is acceptable
(with lunch or dinner, not both!)

Reminders:

❑ One of your fat servings at some point during the day must be either flaxseeds or flax oil.
❑ One of your protein servings at some point during the day must be either fish or soy.
❑ Limit your saturated fat to 20 grams a day if you are healthy; 15 grams if you have an inflammatory or heart condition. You don't need to count the fat found in fish.

What about the treat?

In addition to your meals and snacks, you are allowed one small sweet treat per day at any time of the day you like. Refer to the Gold Coast Foods List on page 183 to see what our definition of "small" is!

Women's Basic Meal Plan for Moderate Activity*

🐵🐵🐵

**Moderate activity includes light daily activity plus a 30- to 35-minute moderate
to high-intensity exercise routine such as our Gold Coast Cure workout.
Several hours of outdoor work, such as light yard work, would also qualify as
moderate activity as long as you are on your feet most of the time.*

Breakfast:

❏ 1 serving fruit

❏ 1 serving dense carbs

❏ 1 serving fat *(any type)*

❏ 1 serving protein *(any type)*

❏ coffee or tea *(if desired)*

Snack:

NOTE: If you don't want to eat a snack, you can incorporate the following
foods into your breakfast, lunch and dinner instead.

❏ 1 serving dense carb *or* 1 serving of either soy or dairy products

❏ ½ serving nuts, seeds or nut butters

❏ 1 serving fruit

Lunch & Dinner:

❏ 1 or 2 servings vegetables

❏ 1½ servings dense carbs

❏ 1 serving fat *(any type)*

❏ 1 serving protein *(any type)*

❏ coffee or tea *(if desired)*

❏ 5 ounces of wine is acceptable

 (with lunch or dinner, not both!)

Reminders:

❏ One of your fat servings at some point during the day must be either
flaxseeds or flax oil.

❏ One of your protein servings at some point during the day must be either
fish or soy.

❏ Limit your saturated fat to 20 grams a day if you are healthy; 15 grams if you
have an inflammatory or heart condition. You don't need to count the fat
found in fish.

What about the treat?

In addition to your meals and snacks, you are allowed one small sweet treat
per day at any time of the day you like. Refer to the Gold Coast Foods List on
page 183 to see what our definition of "small" is!

Women's Basic Meal Plan for the Very Active*

🐒🐒🐒🐒

*Very active includes light daily activity plus a 30- to 35-minute moderate
to high-intensity Gold Coast Cure workout plus an extra 20 to 25 minutes of aerobic
exercise. Alternatively, all-day heavy outdoor labor would qualify as very active.*

Breakfast:

❏ 1 serving fruit   ❏ 1 serving protein *(any type)*
❏ 1 serving dense carbs   ❏ coffee or tea *(if desired)*
❏ 1 serving fat *(any type)*

Snack:

NOTE: If you don't want to eat a snack, you can incorporate the following
foods into your breakfast, lunch and dinner instead.

❏ 1 serving dense carbs
❏ ½ serving nuts, seeds or nut butters
❏ 1 serving fruit
❏ 1 serving of either soy or dairy products

Lunch & Dinner:

❏ 1 or 2 servings vegetables   ❏ coffee or tea *(if desired)*
❏ 1½ servings dense carbs   ❏ 5 ounces of wine is acceptable
❏ 1 serving fat *(any type)*   *(with lunch or dinner, not both!)*
❏ 1 serving protein *(any type)*

Reminders:

❏ One of your fat servings at some point during the day must be either
  flaxseeds or flax oil.
❏ One of your protein servings at some point during the day must be either
  fish or soy.
❏ Limit your saturated fat to 20 grams a day if you are healthy; 15 grams if you
  have an inflammatory or heart condition. You don't need to count the fat
  found in fish.

What about the treat?

In addition to your meals and snacks, you are allowed one small sweet treat
per day at any time of the day you like. Refer to the Gold Coast Foods List on
page 183 to see what our definition of "small" is!

Men's Basic Meal Plan for Very Light Activity*

*Very light activity involves sitting at a desk the majority of the day,
driving a car to work, reading and typing.*

Breakfast:

❑ 1 serving fruit   ❑ 1 serving protein *(any type)*
❑ 2 servings dense carbs   ❑ coffee or tea *(if desired)*
❑ 1 serving fat *(any type)*

Lunch & Dinner:

❑ 1 or 2 servings vegetables   ❑ coffee or tea *(if desired)*
❑ 2 servings dense carbs   ❑ 8 to 10 ounces of wine is acceptable
❑ 1½ servings fat *(any type)*   *(with lunch or dinner, not both!)*
❑ 1 serving protein *(any type)*

Reminders:

❑ One of your fat servings at some point during the day must be either flaxseeds or flax oil.
❑ One of your protein servings at some point during the day must be either fish or soy.
❑ Limit your saturated fat to 20 grams a day if you are healthy; 15 grams if you have an inflammatory or heart condition.

What about the treat?

In addition to your meals and snacks, you are allowed one small sweet treat per day at any time of the day you like. Refer to the Gold Coast Foods List on page 183 to see what our definition of "small" is!

Men's Basic Meal Plan for Light Activity*

🐷🐷

*Light activity would include shopping, running errands, child care, cooking
and light housework. One trip to the grocery store is still very light activity, but several
hours spent shopping or running errands bumps you up into the light category.*

Breakfast:

❑ 1 serving fruit   ❑ 1 serving protein *(any type)*
❑ 2 servings dense carbs   ❑ coffee or tea *(if desired)*
❑ 1 serving fat *(any type)*

Snack:

NOTE: If you don't want to eat a snack, you can incorporate the following
foods into your breakfast, lunch and dinner instead.
❑ 1 serving fruit
❑ 1 serving of either soy or dairy products

Lunch & Dinner:

❑ 1 or 2 servings vegetables   ❑ coffee or tea *(if desired)*
❑ 2 servings dense carbs   ❑ 8 to 10 ounces of wine is acceptable
❑ 1½ servings fat *(any type)*   *(with lunch or dinner, not both!)*
❑ 1 serving protein *(any type)*

Reminders:

❑ One of your fat servings at some point during the day must be either
   flaxseeds or flax oil.
❑ One of your protein servings at some point during the day must be either
   fish or soy.
❑ Limit your saturated fat to 20 grams a day if you are healthy; 15 grams if you
   have an inflammatory or heart condition.

What about the treat?

In addition to your meals and snacks, you are allowed one small sweet treat
per day at any time of the day you like. Refer to the Gold Coast Foods List on
page 183 to see what our definition of "small" is!

Men's Basic Meal Plan for "Moderate" Activity

🐾🐾🐾

*Moderate activity includes light daily activity plus a 30- to 35-minute moderate
to high-intensity exercise routine such as our Gold Coast Cure workout.
Several hours of outdoor work, such as light yard work, would also qualify as
moderate activity as long as you are on your feet most of the time.*

Breakfast:

❑ 1 serving fruit
❑ 2 servings dense carbs
❑ 1 serving fat *(any type)*
❑ 1 serving protein *(any type)*
❑ coffee or tea *(if desired)*

Snack:

NOTE: If you don't want to eat a snack, you can incorporate the following
foods into your breakfast, lunch and dinner instead.

❑ 1 serving fruit
❑ 1 serving of either soy or
dairy products
❑ 1 serving dense carbs
❑ 1 serving nuts, seeds or
nut butters

Lunch & Dinner:

❑ 1 or 2 servings vegetables
❑ 2 servings dense carbs
❑ 1½ servings fat *(any type)*
❑ 1 serving protein *(any type)*
❑ coffee or tea *(if desired)*
❑ 8 to 10 ounces of wine is acceptable
(with lunch or dinner, not both!)

Reminders:

❑ One of your fat servings at some point during the day must be either
flaxseeds or flax oil.
❑ One of your protein servings at some point during the day must be either
fish or soy.
❑ Limit your saturated fat to 20 grams a day if you are healthy; 15 grams if you
have an inflammatory or heart condition. You don't need to count the fat
found in fish.

What about the treat?

In addition to your meals and snacks, you are allowed one small sweet treat
per day at any time of the day you like. Refer to the Gold Coast Foods List on
page 183 to see what our definition of "small" is!

Men's Basic Meal Plan for the Very Active*

🍴🍴🍴🍴

*Very active includes light daily activity plus a 30- to 35-minute moderate
to high-intensity Gold Coast Cure workout plus an extra 20 to 25 minutes of aerobic
exercise. Alternatively, all-day heavy outdoor labor would qualify as very active.*

Breakfast:

❑ 1 serving fruit   ❑ 1 serving protein *(any type)*
❑ 2 servings dense carbs   ❑ coffee or tea *(if desired)*
❑ 1 serving fat *(any type)*

Snack:

NOTE: If you don't want to eat a snack, you can incorporate the following
foods into your breakfast, lunch and dinner instead.

❑ 1 serving of either soy or dairy products
❑ 1 serving dense carbs
❑ 1 serving nuts, seeds or nut butters
❑ 2 servings fruit

Lunch & Dinner:

❑ 1 or 2 servings vegetables   ❑ coffee or tea *(if desired)*
❑ 2 servings dense carbs   ❑ 8 to 10 ounces of wine is acceptable
❑ 1½ servings fat *(any type)*   *(with lunch or dinner, not both!)*
❑ 1 serving protein *(any type)*

Reminders:

❑ One of your fat servings at some point during the day must be either
   flaxseeds or flax oil.
❑ One of your protein servings at some point during the day must be either
   fish or soy.
❑ Limit your saturated fat to 20 grams a day if you are healthy; 15 grams if you
   have an inflammatory or heart condition. You don't need to count the fat
   found in fish.

What about the treat?

In addition to your meals and snacks, you are allowed one small sweet treat
per day at any time of the day you like. Refer to the Gold Coast Foods List on
page 183 to see what our definition of "small" is!

Gold Coast Foods List

This list is broken down into the same categories used in the meal plans provided. All of the whole foods on this list can be eaten as the foundation for your healthy eating plan. For taste variety and for optimal nutrition, try to vary your food choices as much as possible. Our Gold Coast Foods List is intended as a guide only to get you started and is by no means all-inclusive. Use what you've learned in chapters 2 through 5 to add even more variety to your diet.

Carbohydrates

Vegetables

Serving size is not at all important. These are all nutrient-rich low-calorie foods. Eat as many and as much of these foods as you want.

- Artichoke
- Asparagus
- Bell peppers
- Broccoli
- Broccoli rabe
- Brussels sprouts
- Cabbage
- Carrots
- Celery
- Collards
- Eggplant
- Green beans
- Kale
- Leeks
- Mushrooms
- Onions
- Salad greens of any kind, the darker the better
- Snap peas
- Snow peas
- Spinach
- Squash
- Tomatoes
- Tomato sauce
- Zucchini

Fruits

A *fresh* fruit serving is roughly the size of your closed fist, about 1 cup. For dried fruit, one serving is ¼ cup. For fruit juice one serving is 1 cup (we suggest you limit fruit juice if weight management is a problem for you).

- Apples
- Apricots
- Bananas
- Berries *(strawberries, blue-berries, raspberries, boysen-berries, blackberries, etc.)*
- Cantaloupe
- Cherries
- Cranberries
- Dried fruit *(prunes, raisins, apricots, etc.)*
- Fruit juice is acceptable if you are not overweight
- Grapefruit
- Kiwi
- Lemons
- Limes
- Mango
- Nectarines
- Oranges
- Papaya
- Peaches
- Pears
- Pineapple
- Watermelon

Dense Carbs

One serving is equal to ½ cup of cooked grains or cooked pasta, one large slice of whole-grain bread, or ½ cup of beans. These foods are dense in calories, dense in fiber and dense in nutrients, and are designed to be eaten whole. It's perfectly fine to eat somewhat more than the serving size if you desire. Because whole, dense carbohydrates contain fiber, you'll get full and you'll stop eating naturally. If you have no idea what half a cup of food looks like, measure it out several times at first to get an idea. Soon you'll have no problem eye-balling dense carb serving sizes.

- Amaranth
- Brown rice
- Buckwheat
- Bulgur
- Corn
- Cracked wheat
- Kamut
- Millet
- Oats
- Polenta *(whole grain only)*
- Potatoes
- Quinoa
- Rye berries
- Stone-ground corn tortillas
- Stone-ground whole-wheat pita
- Sweet potatoes
- Wheat berries
- Wheat germ
- Whole barley
- Whole-grain bread
  (such as whole wheat)
- Whole-grain crackers
- Whole-grain pasta
  (such as whole wheat)
- Whole wheat
- Whole-wheat couscous
- Wild rice
- Yams

Beans are also considered dense carbs for the purposes of meal planning. One serving is ½ cup.

- Adzuki beans
- Anasazi beans
- Black beans
- Black-eyed peas
- Brown beans
- Cannellini beans
- Chickpeas
- Great Northern beans
- Kidney beans
- Lentils
- Lima beans
- Navy beans
- Peas
- Pinto beans
- Split peas

Proteins

Animal Protein

Always purchase the leanest cuts of meat available. Trim off all visible fat and skin. (Kitchen shears make snipping fat a snap.) Choose white meat chicken and turkey as opposed to dark meat. The fat in animal protein consists mostly of bad saturated fat. *Remember, you do not want to eat more than 15 to 20 grams of saturated fat per day.*

Animal protein serving sizes are easy enough to measure. One animal protein serving is the size and thickness of your palm. We especially like this particular method of "measuring" out meat servings because larger-boned men and women end up eating a larger portion than smaller-boned men and women. The same measuring method applies to chicken, turkey, red meat, pork and game. Try to limit yourself to one serving per day of these foods. If you fill up on meats such as these, it becomes very difficult to get all the servings you need of the even more healthful super-protein foods, fish and soy.

- Beef *(we prefer you choose tenderloin,*
  filet mignon, sirloin or eye of round
  as these are the leanest cuts)
- Chicken
- Lamb
- Pork
- Turkey
- Veal

Eggs

Eggs are in their own category. One serving is two whole eggs. Do not eat more than two eggs (one serving) per day.

Soy

One serving of soy is the size and thickness of your palm. You must eat at least one serving of soy *or* one serving of fish every single day.

- Tofu
- Tempeh
- Textured vegetable protein *(made from soy)*
- Veggie burgers made with soy protein

Use a standard 8-ounce measuring cup to determine serving size for these soy products.

- Edamame beans *(½ cup is one serving)*
- Soy milk *(1 cup is one serving)*
- Shredded veggie cheese *(½ cup is one serving)*
- Soy nuts, also known as "dry roasted soybeans" *(¼ cup is one serving)*
- Soy chili *(½ cup is one serving)*

Fish

Again, you can use your palm size and palm thickness to estimate a single serving of the following foods. Remember to eat at least one serving of soy or one serving of fish every day.

- Clams
- Crab
- Dolphin *(mahi mahi)*
- Flounder
- Grouper
- Halibut
- Lobster
- Orange roughy
- Oysters
- Shrimp
- Snapper
- Tilapia

Certain fatty fish *must* be eaten in order to enjoy Gold Coast health. These are some of nature's best sources of omega-3 fat. You should choose to eat these particular fish *at least* twice per week. Once again, use your palm size and palm thickness to estimate a single serving of the following foods.

- Anchovy
- Black cod
- Salmon
- Sardines

- Bluefin tuna   • Sea bass
- Herring   • Striped bass
- Mackerel   • Trout
- Sablefish   • White *(albacore)* tuna

Dairy Products

One serving is one 8-ounce cup of the following foods.

- Low-fat milk
- Low-fat yogurt or kefir *(no sugar added)*

Cheese is a bit trickier to measure. Since low-fat cheese has less saturated fat than full-fat cheese, you can eat twice as much.

- Full-fat cheese *(one serving is ¼ cup shredded cheese)*
- Low-fat cheese *(one serving is ½ cup shredded cheese)*

Fats

Nuts, Seeds and Nut Butters

One serving of nuts or seeds is equal to 2 heaping tablespoons. One serving of nut butter is 1 tablespoon. Avoid nuts and seeds that have been roasted in oil. Only purchase raw nuts or dry-roasted nuts.

- Sesame seeds, dry roasted or raw
- Sunflower seeds, dry roasted or raw
- Pumpkin seeds, dry roasted or raw
- Almonds or all-natural almond butter *(to repeat, all-natural means no hydrogenated oils and no partially hydrogenated oils, period)*
- Cashews or all-natural cashew nut butter
- Chestnuts
- Hazelnuts or all-natural hazelnut butter

- Peanuts or all-natural peanut butter
- Pecans
- Pine nuts
- Pistachios
- Tahini *(sesame seed butter)*
- Walnuts

Oils and Fatty Condiments

For all oils one serving is 1 tablespoon.

- Extra-virgin olive oil, use for either no-heat or high-heat recipes
- Extra-virgin coconut oil, use for either no-heat or high-heat recipes
- High-oleic canola oil, use for cooking
- Expeller-pressed canola oil, use for no-heat recipes
- High-oleic safflower oil, use for cooking
- High-oleic sunflower oil, use for cooking
- Flax oil, use for no-heat recipes

Fatty condiments have variable serving sizes.

- Avocado, ¼ of an avocado equals one serving
- Butter, one serving is 1 tablespoon
- Canola-oil based mayonnaise, 1 tablespoon is one serving
- Flaxseeds, one serving is equal to 3 tablespoons ground flaxseeds
- Olives, 15 small olives is one serving
- Hummus, ¼ cup is one serving. Be sure the hummus you buy is made with either olive oil or expeller-pressed canola oil

Your Daily Sweet Treat

It is acceptable to include one small treat or dessert as part of your daily meal plan if desired. Overweight individuals will enjoy quicker weight loss if they skip these treats entirely—no surprises here. No matter how much you weigh, it's important from a health standpoint to eat no more than one small dessert each day. If you're too thin and you need to gain weight, add more healthy nutrient-rich foods, not more sweets.

If all you really need is the taste of something sweet after your meal, try a few bites of dried fruit, nuts or even a small bit of a high-quality all-natural dark chocolate before reaching for sugar-laden, empty-calorie sweet treats if at all possible.

We define "sweet treat" desserts as sweet-tasting foods made primarily from sugar and flour. These foods often contain all-natural sources of saturated fat such as eggs, milk and butter. Desserts may contain sugar, cream, alcohol, butter and flour. They can, and should, also contain nuts and fruit whenever possible. Just remember, Gold Coast Cure desserts absolutely must be *all-natural*; they may *never* contain the "Red Light" trans fats found in margarine, hydrogenated oil, partially hydrogenated oil or vegetable shortening.

Obviously the vast majority of desserts contain a significant amount of sugar. One of the easiest and tastiest ways to reduce the sugar (and calorie) content of your desserts is to make them at home using Splenda as a substitute for at least *some* of the sugar. As long as you don't replace more than about half of the sugar in any given recipe with Splenda, you'll absolutely not notice any difference in either taste or texture.

Many desserts are made with refined, enriched flour. If you choose to make your desserts at home, why not make them a bit more healthful by using at least a little bit of whole-wheat flour in place of refined flour? A sample list of acceptable, all-natural desserts follows.

- Homemade or all-natural cookies
- All-natural ice cream
- Good quality dark chocolate made without hydrogenated or partially hydrogenated oil
- Mousse
- Bread puddings
- Sweet (dessert) wines
- Sweet liqueurs, ports, brandies, sherries
- Custards
- Pastries made without vegetable shortening

- Soufflé
- Cakes made without vegetable shortening
- Cheesecake
- Crème brûlée
- Fruit crisp or fruit pie

We allow a small dessert each day because total deprivation is neither fun nor realistic. A little sweet treat is not going to ruin your health. However, "little" is a relative term, especially when it comes to dessert. It's important to be clear here. As a general rule of thumb, rich desserts such as cheesecake, crème brûlée, brownie, pie or cake should be no larger than about 1 inch thick and half the size of your palm (not including your thumb and fingers). Servings of ice cream, puddings, mousse and soufflé should be no larger than ½ cup, 4 ounces. Lighter desserts made with fruit and flour only and containing a minimal amount of fat or cream such as apple crisp can be about 1 inch thick and the size of your palm, but no more!

Menus

The Cure is easy to follow because we put you in the driver's seat. On your way, though, a map can be helpful. The following menus were created using the Women's Basic Meal Plan for Moderate Activity. Please note the meal plans are a *guideline* only. For example, if you're a very active woman or man, you'll need to eat more food than what we suggest below.

As you'll see, following the Cure is not about starvation or denial. The menu suggestions are simple to follow and satisfying, and they'll ease you into the Gold Coast mind-set. After a few days of following the Cure's meal plans, creating balanced meals from healthy whole foods will be like second nature.

Day: 1

BREAKFAST:

1 cup Nature's Path Organic Flax Plus Multigrain Cereal with
  1 tablespoon flaxseeds
  1 cup soy milk
  Sliced fresh strawberries

Coffee with all-natural half and half cream *or* green tea with soy milk

LUNCH:

½ cup black bean chili *(such as Amy's Medium Black Bean Chili)*

Stone-ground corn tortilla topped with ¼ cup melted Monterey Jack cheese

Side salad of mixed greens and 2 tablespoons sunflower seeds
  Dress with flax oil and lemon juice

SNACK:

Yogurt and fruit parfait

Combine 1 cup low-fat, no-sugar-added yogurt with 2 tablespoons chopped
  walnuts and ¾ cup fresh fruit of your choosing *(raspberries, blueberries,
  peaches, etc.)*

DINNER:

Filet mignon

Wheat berry pilaf

Spinach sautéed with extra-virgin olive oil and garlic

1 glass of wine *(optional)*

Optional Sweet Treat: ½ cup-scoop all-natural vanilla ice cream topped with
  fresh strawberries and chocolate sauce

Day: 2

BREAKFAST:

1 slice Nutty Carrot Raisin Bread *(Gold Coast recipe)* topped with 1 teaspoon
  Smart Balance Omega Plus spread

1 hard-boiled egg

1 cup sliced oranges

Coffee with all-natural half and half cream *or* green tea with soy milk

LUNCH:

Sandwich on two pieces toasted whole-grain bread with:
- Ham *(2 or 3 medium slices)*
- Low-fat cheese *(1 slice)*
- Tomato slices
- Spinach or dark salad greens
- 1 or 2 teaspoons canola-oil mayonnaise

Carrot and celery sticks dipped in either hummus *or* Lemon Cashew Dip *(Gold Coast recipe)*

SNACK:

1 ounce *(¼ cup)* low-fat cheese with 1 serving whole-grain crackers

Fresh peach

DINNER:

Baked salmon with fish rub *(such as Emeril's Fish Rub)*

¾ cup whole-wheat couscous

Side salad of mixed greens dressed with fresh lemon juice and flax oil

1 glass of wine *(optional)*

Optional Sweet Treat: Mixed berries topped with 1 tablespoon all-natural fresh whipped cream

---

Day: 3

BREAKFAST:

Omelet prepared with two eggs and one finely chopped red pepper
    Sauté the pepper in 1 teaspoon extra-virgin olive oil

1 cup pineapple chunks

1 piece whole grain toast topped with 1 teaspoon whipped butter

Coffee with milk *or* green tea with soy milk

LUNCH:

1 cup split pea soup *(such as Amy's Split Pea Soup)* topped with ¼ cup soy cheese

1 serving *(about 15 chips)* of health-food quality tortilla chips *(such as Garden of Eatin' Black Bean Tortilla Chips)*

Fresh salsa

SNACK:

5 *or* 6 flax crackers *(such as Dr. Kracker Classic 3 Seed)* or other whole-grain cracker

1 cup soy milk

DINNER:

Spiced Pork Chops with Apple Onion Compote *(Gold Coast recipe)*

Mashed sweet potatoes made using either Smart Balance *or* Earth Balance spread

Green beans with slivered almonds

1 glass of wine *(optional)*

Optional Sweet Treat: Paradise Prune Squares with Lemon Cream Cheese Frosting *(Gold Coast recipe)*

Day: 4

BREAKFAST:

1 serving No-Fuss Baked Banana French Toast Casserole *(Gold Coast recipe; contains flaxseeds)* topped with 1 tablespoon all-natural nut butter of choice

Coffee with milk *or* green tea with soy milk

LUNCH:

Mixed salad greens served with:
  • Shredded carrots
  • 1 tablespoon Amazing Apple Vinaigrette *(Gold Coast recipe)* or any other store-bought all-natural vinaigrette of your choosing. Try Annie's Naturals Cilantro & Lime Vinaigrette, for example.

Veggie Pita Pizza Sandwich
  Fill whole-wheat pita bread with the following, then heat briefly in your microwave until the cheese melts:
  • ¼ cup all-natural marinara sauce *(try Amy's brand)*
  • Fresh spinach leaves
  • ½ cup low-fat shredded cheese

Salt and pepper to taste

SNACK:

Baked apple with ¼ cup melted low-fat cheddar cheese *or* 2 tablespoons walnuts

DINNER:

Parsley & Nut-Crusted Baked Halibut *(Gold Coast recipe)*

Asparagus with extra-virgin olive oil

Corn on the cob with a pat of Smart Balance *or* Earth Balance spread

1 glass of wine *(optional)*

Optional Sweet Treat: Almond Apricot Bread Pudding *(Gold Coast recipe)*

Day: 5

BREAKFAST:

1 slice whole-grain bread topped with 1 teaspoon peanut butter

1 cup low-fat yogurt topped with ½ cup mixed berries, 2 tablespoons flaxseeds; sweeten with Splenda *or* stevia to taste

Coffee with all-natural half and half cream *or* green tea with soy milk

LUNCH:

Quick Green Bean Salad *(thaw frozen green beans and season with balsamic vinegar, flaxseed oil, salt and pepper)*

Oat bran pita stuffed with either tuna salad *or* egg salad

    Tuna salad or egg salad can be made using:

- ½ cup canned tuna *(or 1 hardboiled whole egg plus 1 egg white)*
- 1 tablespoon canola oil mayonnaise
- ¼ cup celery, finely chopped
- 1 thinly sliced scallion *(optional)*
- Dried dill, to taste
- Salt and pepper to taste

SNACK:

Banana and Peanut Butter Smoothie

    Combine 1 tablespoon all-natural peanut butter, 1 cup soy milk, 1 banana, 1 packet Splenda sweetener, and 3 ice cubes in the blender, then whip until smooth

DINNER:

Parisian Vegetable Beef Stew *(Gold Coast recipe)*

Mixed salad greens topped with roasted red peppers and 2 tablespoons sunflower seeds

1 glass of wine *(optional)*

Optional Sweet Treat: Apple-Spice Crisp *(Gold Coast recipe)*

Day: 6

BREAKFAST:

1 cup fresh mixed fruit

Breakfast sandwich

Grill together on a skillet in 1 teaspoon extra-virgin olive oil:
- 2 slices whole-grain toast
- 1 tomato, sliced
- 1 slice low-fat cheese

Coffee with all-natural half and half cream *or* green tea with soy milk

LUNCH:

Poached salmon

Fresh spinach salad dressed with Honey Lovin' Lime Vinaigrette
(Gold Coast recipe)

¾ cup frozen corn kernels mixed with ¼ cup salsa and 1 teaspoon extra-virgin
olive oil

SNACK:

1 cup low-fat plain kefir

3 tablespoons flaxseeds

½ cup fresh raspberries

DINNER:

Roasted chicken

Bistro Style Oven-Roasted Veggies & Potatoes *(Gold Coast recipe)*

1 glass of wine *(optional)*

Optional Sweet Treat: Baked apple, cored, stuffed with ½ cup of all-natural
vanilla ice cream and 2 tablespoons chopped walnuts

Day: 7

BREAKFAST:

Apple slices

½ of a sprouted whole-wheat toasted bagel topped with 1 tablespoon all-natural
whipped cream cheese and 2 ounces smoked salmon *(lox)*

Coffee with milk *or* green tea with soy milk

LUNCH:

Thickly sliced tomatoes topped with sliced fresh buffalo mozzarella drizzled with balsamic vinegar and flax oil

1 cup bean soup *(such as Coco Pazzo Tuscan Five Bean Soup with Barley)*

SNACK:

1 cup low-fat latte sweetened with Splenda *or* stevia

Trail Mix

Combine 2 tablespoons sunflower seeds with 1 tablespoon semi-sweet dark chocolate chips *(try the gourmet Ghirardelli Double Chocolate brand)* and 2 tablespoons raisins

DINNER:

Arugula and fresh mozzarella salad dressed with balsamic vinegar and flax oil

Lemon Roasted Scallops with Artichokes *(Gold Coast recipe)*

Barley seasoned with extra-virgin olive oil

1 glass of wine *(optional)*

Optional Sweet Treat: Luscious Pumpkin Cheesecake *(Gold Coast recipe)*

Day: 8

BREAKFAST:

Blender shake made with 1 cup soy milk, 1 banana, 3 ice cubes, 1 teaspoon almond butter, 3 tablespoons ground flaxseeds; sweeten with Splenda *or* stevia to taste

LUNCH:

Bean burrito

Wrap the following in a whole-grain tortilla such as Food for Life's Ezekiel 4:9 Sprouted Grain Tortillas, then heat briefly in the microwave:
- ½ cup pinto beans, mashed or whole
- ¼ cup low-fat cheddar cheese
- 1 tablespoon all-natural guacamole
- Shredded carrots
- Finely chopped onions

1 cup gazpacho *or* fresh tomato salsa

SNACK:

1 tablespoon almond butter on a whole-grain cracker

Apple

1 cup soy milk

DINNER:

1 cup whole-wheat pasta

½ cup prepared marinara sauce *(such as Victoria Marinara)*

3 prepared meatless meatballs *(such as Nate's Savory Mushroom Meatless Meatballs)*

2 tablespoons Parmesan cheese

1 glass of wine *(optional)*

Optional Sweet Treat: 1 small square *(1 inch)* dark gourmet chocolate

Day: 9

BREAKFAST:

1 glass low-fat milk

1 Chunky Apple-Raisin Morning Muffin *(Gold Coast recipe)* topped with 2 teaspoons nut butter

Coffee with all-natural half and half cream *or* green tea with soy milk

LUNCH:

¾ cup tabbouleh *(look for this Middle Eastern salad in your supermarket's deli)*

Rotisserie chicken breast *(can also be found in your supermarket's deli)*

½ of a whole-wheat pita bread with 2 tablespoons hummus

1 cup fresh strawberries

SNACK:

½ cup low-fat cottage cheese

3 tablespoons flaxseeds

½ cup blueberries

DINNER:

Far Eastern Tofu & Vegetable Stir Fry *(Gold Coast recipe)*

¾ cup long-grain brown rice

1 glass of wine *(optional)*

Optional Sweet Treat: Chocolate Brownie Apple Nut Cake *(Gold Coast recipe)*

Day: 10

BREAKFAST:

Hot cereal

Mix the following ingredients, then heat in the microwave for 1½ minutes:
- ½ cup old-fashioned oatmeal
- 3 tablespoons ground flaxseeds
- ¾ cup low-fat milk *or* soy milk
- Sweeten with Splenda *or* stevia to taste
  Top with fresh raspberries

Coffee with all-natural half and half cream *or* green tea with soy milk

LUNCH:

Chicken, feta cheese and roasted pepper roll-up sandwich
- Use a sprouted whole-grain tortilla
- To make this meal in a hurry, purchase pre-roasted red peppers and pre-cooked chicken breasts from your grocery store deli
- Use ¼ cup "light" feta cheese

Add a side salad of baby spinach or mixed green lettuce leaves

Top with a vinaigrette dressing made from balsamic vinegar and either flax oil *or* extra-virgin olive oil

SNACK:

1 cup high-fiber cereal *(such as Barbara's Bakery Multigrain Shredded Spoonfuls)*

½ cup soy milk *or* low-fat milk

DINNER:

Lime-Marinated Sea Bass with Chili-Spice Rub *(Gold Coast recipe)*

Broccoli rabe sautéed in extra-virgin olive oil

¾ cup lentils seasoned with garlic and extra-virgin olive oil

1 glass of wine *(optional)*

Optional Sweet Treat: Fresh berries topped with ½ cup of all-natural chocolate ice cream

Day: 11

BREAKFAST:

1 cup Kashi GOLEAN brand cold cereal topped with 1 cup low-fat milk *or* soy milk, 2 tablespoons sunflower seeds, fresh raspberries

Coffee with all-natural half and half cream *or* green tea with soy milk

LUNCH:

1 cup Manhattan clam chowder *(or Gold Coast Clam Chowder, recipe)*

½ cup frozen butter beans with 1 teaspoon butter

Arugula salad with flaxseed oil and balsamic vinegar

SNACK:

1 slice Nutty Carrot Raisin Bread *(Gold Coast recipe)*

1 cup low-fat milk

DINNER:

Curried Apple-Turkey Burgers *(Gold Coast recipe)* topped with avocado slices, served on a whole grain bun

Fresh tomato salad drizzled with flaxseed oil and balsamic vinegar

1 glass of wine *(optional)*

Optional Sweet Treat: Lemony Pecan Bites *(Gold Coast recipe)*

Day: 12

BREAKFAST:

Dutch-Apple Pancakes *(Gold Coast recipe; contains ½ serving flaxseeds)* topped with 2 tablespoons chopped walnuts and 1 or 2 teaspoons of real maple syrup

Coffee with all-natural half and half cream *or* green tea with soy milk

LUNCH:

Stuffed baked potato

Prebake a small potato at 400 degrees for 1 hour. Poke holes in the potato before baking. Bake *without* wrapping your potato in tin foil. Stuff your potato with one item from each of the following three columns:

PROTEIN	FAT	VEGETABLE
Hard-boiled egg *(chopped)*	Chopped olives	Steamed broccoli *(chopped)*
Cottage cheese	Roasted garlic *(with oil)*	Marinara sauce

Shredded low-fat cheese	Low-fat sour cream	Roasted red peppers *(chopped)*
Tofu- *or* turkey-based chili	Pesto	Shredded carrots
Canadian bacon	Guacamole	Fresh tomato salsa

SNACK:

Carrot sticks dipped in ¼ cup all-natural hummus

DINNER:

Garlicky Tomato Shrimp *(Gold Coast recipe)*

½ cup frozen petite peas with 1 teaspoon butter

¾ cup whole-wheat couscous drizzled with 1 teaspoon flaxseed oil

1 glass of wine *(optional)*

Optional Sweet Treat: 1 cookie *(such as Country Choice Peanut Butter Cookie)*

Day: 13

BREAKFAST:

1 slice *(1-inch thick)* Nature's Path Carrot Raisin Manna Bread topped with 1 teaspoon Smart Balance Omega Plus spread

1 hard-boiled egg

1 cup of grapes

Coffee with all-natural half and half cream *or* green tea with soy milk

LUNCH:

Salad of mixed greens with flax oil vinaigrette

1 cup of frozen corn kernels topped with 1 teaspoon Earth Balance *or* Smart Balance spread

Veggie or tofu burger topped with ¼ cup low-fat cheese *(cook veggie burger in the microwave)*

1 cup of sliced watermelon

SNACK:

Granola cereal *(such as Zoe Foods Honey Almond Flax & Soy Granola Cereal)*

1 cup low-fat milk

DINNER:

Grilled lamb loin chops

Potato fries *(such as Alexia Oven Fries with Olive Oil, Rosemary, and Garlic)*

Mixed Salad Greens with Pear and Feta Cheese *(Gold Coast recipe)*

1 glass of wine *(optional)*

Optional Sweet Treat: Fresh cherries drizzled with 2 tablespoons hot chocolate
sauce *(melt 2 ounces dark gourmet chocolate in the microwave with
1 tablespoon light cream)* and 2 tablespoons pistachios

Day: 14

BREAKFAST:

½ cup low-fat cottage cheese mixed with 2 tablespoons wheat germ, ½ cup
fresh or frozen pitted cherries, splash of vanilla extract *(optional)*; sweeten
with Splenda *or* stevia to taste

1 slice whole-grain toast topped with 1 teaspoon almond butter

Coffee with all-natural half and half cream *or* green tea with soy milk

LUNCH:

Caesar's Salad *(Gold Coast recipe; contains flaxseed oil)* plus:
Sliced chicken breast (can be bought from deli section of grocery store)
Whole-grain roll dipped in 1 teaspoon flaxseed oil and 1 tablespoon shaved
Parmesan cheese

Sliced strawberries

SNACK:

1 slice Nature's Path Fruit and Nut Manna Bread *(a delicious fiber-rich sweet
bread made without any sugar!)*

1 teaspoon all-natural nut butter of choice

DINNER:

Frozen pizza (such as A.C. LaRocco Cheese and Garlic Pizza)

Fresh spinach salad with shredded carrots and Annie's Naturals Roasted Red
Pepper Vinaigrette

1 glass of wine *(optional)*

Optional Sweet Treat: One slice marble cake make using Dr. Oetker Marble
Cake Baking Mix

A School Week's Worth of
Kids' Healthy Lunch Box Ideas

Day 1

Ham and cheese *(use low-fat cheese)* sandwich on whole-wheat bread
  (use canola oil mayonnaise)
Grapes
Nutty Dessert Topping *(Gold Coast recipe)*
Boxed long-life soymilk *(such as Eden Soy)* or low-fat milk *(such as
  Parmalat)*
NOTE: *If you freeze the milk, it will be cold at lunchtime*

Day 2

Peanut butter (use all-natural only) and jelly on whole-grain bread
Carrot sticks dipped in Lemon Cashew Dip *(Gold Coast recipe)*
Pitted cherries
Boxed long-life soymilk *(such as Eden Soy)* or low-fat milk
  (such as Parmalat)
NOTE: *If you freeze the milk, it will be cold at lunchtime*

Day 3

Ants on a Log *(stuff celery with all-natural peanut butter and top with
  raisins)*
Dole Fruit Bowls Pineapple *(this variety contains no added sugary syrups)*
Low-fat string cheese
Whole-wheat crackers
Hardboiled egg
Boxed long-life low-fat chocolate milk *(such as Parmalat)*
NOTE: *If you freeze the milk, it will be cold at lunchtime*

Day 4

Cheese *(use low-fat cheese)* sandwich on whole-grain bread
  (use canola oil mayonnaise)
Granola bar *(such as Nature Valley)* or trail mix bar *(such as Save the
  Forest Organic Trail Mix Bars)*
Apple
Bottled water

Day 5
Nutty Carrot Raisin Bread *(Gold Coast recipe)*
$\frac{1}{2}$ of a tuna fish sandwich *(made with canola oil mayonnaise and sweet relish)* on whole-grain bread
Fresh strawberries
Low-fat cheese cubes
Bottled water

Dining Out

You can eat out, enjoy yourself *and* eat healthfully if you take a few precautions. It's usually easier to eat healthfully at higher-quality restaurants because they tend to use fresher ingredients and include healthier items on their menu. The waiters also tend to be more willing to make adjustments. We're not saying you can only dine at the best of the best while on the Cure, but be aware that you often get what you pay for. For example, it's much cheaper for the restaurant to serve a huge mound of white pasta than it is to serve the same size portion of vegetables. Lower-end restaurants are notorious for serving enormous portions of empty-calorie foods such as white pasta and bread. Many people think these huge portions represent a fabulous deal. This is absolutely not the case. White pasta and white bread are ridiculously inexpensive for restaurants to purchase and mark up.

When eating out, remember to order balanced meals that include vegetables, a moderate amount of protein, good fats, and nutrient- and fiber-rich dense carbohydrates. You don't have to clean your plate. Most restaurants serve enormous portions. Doggy bags still exist, so don't be shy about asking for one.

The Dos and Don'ts of Eating Out

1) Don't eat the bread! Unless specifically stated otherwise assume all restaurant bread is made from enriched flour as opposed to

whole grains. This rule applies even at the finest restaurants. For this reason, sandwiches are not a good choice unless you skip the bread. Remember, breads made with refined flour contain no nutrients. Many contain deadly trans fats.

2) Avoid all fried foods when dining out, period.

3) Order salads, either as an appetizer or your entrée. If you choose a salad as your main entrée, be sure to add proteins such as chicken, fish or eggs; fats such as avocado or olives; and a side of healthful nutrient-rich carbohydrates such as beans, potatoes, sweet potatoes or corn. Salads are one of your best restaurant picks because you can add so many healthful foods and you have control over your meal because you can see all the ingredients. Always ask for your salad dressing on the side, and always stick to the vinaigrettes as opposed to the creamy dressings. You can also request extra-virgin olive oil, balsamic vinegar and lemon juice on the side.

More salad tips:

- Add vegetables. If the salad you want doesn't come with enough vegetables, scan the menu, see what vegetables are offered elsewhere, and request those on your salad or as a side.
- Add protein. Go for grilled chicken, hard-boiled eggs, grilled calamari, shrimp, seared tuna or steak strips.
- Keep cheese portions small because most restaurants don't offer low-fat cheese. However, a little cheese adds a lot of flavor and satisfaction to any salad. Parmesan cheese is a good choice with only 4 grams of saturated fat per ¼ cup. Feta cheese is another good choice.
- Add nuts, seeds, olives or avocado. These good fats keep you feeling full. You may even want to consider bringing your own nuts and seeds in with you.
- If you are at a salad bar, look for beans, corn or peas.

4) Choose a bean dish. Look for black bean or split pea soup. Hummus is another great restaurant food. Request a side dish of beans to replace unhealthful standard sides such as white rice, French fries, or buttery, skinless mashed potatoes.

5) Soup is another good choice. Try bean-based soups, miso soup, onion soups served without the bread and cheese, vegetable soups, Manhattan clam chowder or gazpacho. Avoid creamy and pasta-based soups.

6) Order seafood. Fish, lobster, shrimp, calamari and scallop dishes are great choices. Ask that your seafood be cooked with as little butter as possible. Alternatively, tell the waiter you're on a special diet and the only oil you can have is olive oil. Avoid cream sauces or ask for them on the side, and use only a smidgen. No fried seafood!

7) Chicken, turkey and lean beef are also good choices as long as they aren't fried or smothered with sauces. Avoid hamburgers when eating out. Most restaurants offer the fattiest, cheapest burgers possible. Ribs are a terrible choice, too, prime rib included.

8) Baked potatoes served with the skin, corn, beans, tabbouleh and fresh fruit are good, nutrient-rich carbohydrate choices. If you're eating breakfast, ask for oatmeal.

9) Always order a side dish of vegetables. Request that they be steamed or cooked in extra-virgin olive oil if possible. A *small* amount of butter is acceptable as a second choice.

10) Ask for all sauces on the side and go easy with your serving size. Avoid creamy sauces—these are often loaded with saturated fat at high-quality restaurants, and either processed vegetable oil or even trans fats at family-style restaurants. Standard marinara-style sauces make a safe, healthful choice if you don't want to trouble the waiter too much.

11) Avoid pasta dishes when dining out. Save pasta for home-cooked meals when you can use the whole-grain version. Besides, there are far more interesting foods to order when dining out.

12) Avoid breaded meats, chickens and fishes, even if they are baked. That means no seafood cakes.

13) No standard sodas. No sweetened tea. No lemonade. Unsweetened iced tea, seltzers and water are far better choices.

14) A glass or two of wine is your best alcoholic beverage choice. Women should stick to one glass except on special occasions. A glass of beer every now and then is also fine, but wine is better. If you absolutely must have hard liquor, order the driest drink possible. Steer clear of sweet "umbrella" drinks such as margaritas, rum punches, flavored martinis and piña coladas.

15) Seek out simply prepared foods rather than complicated recipes. The more complicated the recipe, the more likely it is to include unhealthful ingredients. For example, if you order tuna tartare, you can see exactly what it is you're eating, tuna and spice! If you order crab cakes, you have absolutely no idea what you're putting into your mouth.

16) Desserts must be small. Obviously fresh fruit is your best bet, but we admit that plain old fruit might be a bit boring. A *small* serving of something really fabulous, perhaps homemade cheesecake, is acceptable if you've eaten a well-balanced meal.

17) Coffee and tea are also fine. Avoid adding sugar and avoid artificial whiteners containing vegetable oils and trans fats. Use milk rather than cream.

Now that you've learned the secret to healthful meal planning, the next chapter explains the Gold Coast philosophy of maximum fitness in minimum time.

10 Gold Coast Fitness: Maximum Results, Minimum Time

A good diet alone is not enough to keep you healthy. Only by combining a sensible food plan with a consistent fitness program can you obtain optimal health. However, unless you happen to be a professional athlete dependent upon physical fitness for your income or a truly dedicated sports enthusiast, you probably want to enjoy the absolute minimum amount of fitness "fun."

A problem with many fitness programs is that they require tremendous time commitment. For those of us who don't enjoy spending time at the gym—or simply don't have time to go to a gym—the Gold Coast fitness routine is a blessing. This chapter is all about discovering shortcuts to achieving the fit body you desire

The best-kept secret in exercise science—resistance circuit-training— is the workout program guaranteed to get you fittest fastest. The custom resistance circuit-training exercise routine we present at the end of this chapter will get you into shape and keep you in shape with less than two hours per week of effort. The surprising truth is 90 percent of the health benefits that can be obtained from exercise can be achieved with approximately two hours per week of effort. The best part is, you don't even have to leave your house unless you want to.

There are very few chronic diseases that don't benefit from exercise. Studies have proven that exercise significantly reduces the severity of many common medical conditions. Here's just a partial list of what exercise can do for you:

- Lower your blood pressure.[1]
- Improve your lung function. If you have asthma, this is especially important.
- Improve your cholesterol profile.[2]
- Prevent and even *reverse* osteoporosis.[3]
- Decrease the pain associated with arthritis.[4]
- Improve the symptoms of fibromyalgia.[5]
- Decrease rates of depression, anxiety and stress.
- Improve your energy levels if you suffer from chronic fatigue syndrome.[6]
- Reduce your risk of cancer.[7]
- Prevent or reverse the course of type 2 diabetes by increasing your body's ability to tolerate more carbohydrates without an increase in your blood sugar level and without an increase in insulin secretion.[8]
- Improve strength, balance and coordination of those with MS.

Just for Diabetics: Why You *Really Need* to Exercise

If you have diabetes, increasing your muscle mass through resistance training exercises can help you reduce or even eliminate your need for insulin shots and sugar pills. Large, active muscles "eat" sugar, and they need very little insulin to do so. In other words, having muscle mass lowers your blood sugar level without insulin. As soon as your need to inject the "fat-storing" hormone insulin decreases, fat loss becomes possible and your health will dramatically improve.

During your actual exercise session, the picture is even brighter. Blood sugar levels and blood insulin levels stay low when you exercise, and during and immediately following exercise sugar is taken out of your bloodstream and absorbed by your muscles much faster than normal. It takes a scant amount of insulin for actively exercising muscles to absorb and burn off blood sugar. When you perform resistance circuit-training exercises, you keep your blood sugar at a healthy, low level despite producing almost no insulin at all.

What Overweight Nondiabetics Need to Know

Even if you're not diabetic and you don't have insulin resistance, you're not out of the woods if you're overweight. Inactive, overweight people have muscles that are filled to the brim with glycogen, a storage form of sugar energy. If you're overweight and you eat more carbohydrates or protein than necessary, your blood sugar level spikes. The *only* difference between you and a diabetic is that you can still produce enough insulin to keep your blood sugar level from getting dangerously high. However, while the insulin your body produces succeeds in lowering your blood sugar level, this insulin still ends up causing harm in the long run. Because your muscles are already full of glycogen, your leftover blood sugar energy has nowhere to go except to your liver, an organ that converts sugar into fat. This fat is then transported to fat cells for storage on your stomach, thighs and butt.

Exercise will give you "hungry" active muscles that will defeat this vicious cycle.

Debunking Three Popular Fitness Myths

Fitness, like nutrition, is often misunderstood. A lot of people either have no idea how to get into shape, or worse, they have developed erroneous notions about what it takes to get fit and stay fit. Before you hop on the nearest treadmill in an attempt to lose weight, read this section! You'll soon understand why "treadmill only" fitness programs get you nowhere fast.

Myth #1: Dieting works just as well as exercise for weight-loss purposes.

Drastically reducing your calorie intake without exercising is *not* the way to go if lasting weight loss is your goal because dieting causes you to lose both fat and muscle. Low-calorie diets slow down your resting metabolic rate and make weight management significantly more difficult in the long run. Muscle is lean, metabolically active tissue you can't afford to lose. When you lose weight on a low-calorie diet, up to 30 percent of the weight you lose comes from metabolically active muscle. If, for example, you "successfully" drop 15 pounds on a low-calorie diet, as many as 4½ of those pounds come from muscle. The more weight you lose on a low-calorie diet, the more damage you cause to your metabolism. For example, if you lose 4½ pounds of muscle you have to eat 180 calories less every single day to maintain your weight loss. If you lose 6½ pounds of muscle you have to eat 260 calories less every single day to maintain your weight loss. On a low-calorie diet, your weight loss tends to eventually plateau as your metabolism slows down, while at the same time your sense of food and nutrient deprivation increases. This is a bad combination.

If, on the other hand, you manage to lose weight while *increasing* your muscle mass through resistance exercise, your metabolic rate can actually *increase* despite weight loss.[9] The only way to increase your metabolism as you lose weight is to build up your muscles by performing resistance training exercises such as the workout we provide later in this chapter.

The secret to permanent weight loss is to gradually reduce your calorie intake by following a filling, nutrient-rich, whole-foods diet while simultaneously performing the Cure's 30 minutes of resistance circuit-training exercise three times a week to build metabolically active muscle and therefore increase your metabolic rate. Dieting alone is not optimally effective.

Myth #2: Aerobic exercise is the best exercise for fat loss.

Take a look at what happens if you spend a total of 90 minutes every week exercising and you choose from among the following workouts.

All of the following calculations are based on a sample 150-pound adult woman.

At the end of one year if you are over age 35:

- As a fitness walker you would lose 5½ pounds.
- As a runner or cyclist you would lose 13½ pounds.
- As a Gold Coast exerciser you would lose 23½ pounds.

1) Walking

Walking at the brisk pace of 15 minutes per mile for 30 minutes three times a week, a 150-pound person would burn a total of 504 calories at the end of the week. Although fitness walking does strengthen your cardiovascular system, walking does not increase metabolically active muscle and walking does not prevent the muscle atrophy associated with aging. Nevertheless, burning an extra 504 calories every week results in a loss of 7½ pounds of fat over the course of an entire year.

Unfortunately, there is a slight catch if you're over the age of 35. After age 35 you lose about a half pound of muscle each year unless you perform some type of resistance exercise. If you lose this muscle you will gain 2 pounds of fat each year unless you reduce your calorie intake with each birthday. Why would you gain this weight? With a half pound of missing muscle, your metabolism would slow by 20 calories every day. This adds up to 7,300 extra calories every year, the equivalent of 2 pounds of fat. All told, if you are over age 35, you end up losing only 5½ pounds in the first year of your 90 minutes weekly fitness walking program. Good, but far from ideal.

The best thing we can say about fitness walking is most people can indeed walk briskly for the full 30 minutes three times a week. Unfortunately, that is not the case with our next example.

2) Running or Cycling

Running at 6 miles per hour and cycling at 15 miles per hour are two activities that burn lots of calories in a short amount of time. The problem is, few adults, even reasonably fit adults, can bicycle or run for 30 minutes straight at these speeds. Besides, huffing and puffing to exhaustion is not something we find particularly enjoyable.

Nevertheless, let's pretend our 150-pound adult is fit and therefore capable of performing high-intensity aerobic exercise. At the end of one week, a runner or cyclist exercising for a total of 90 minutes would burn 1,044 calories. By the end of the year this runner or cyclist would lose 15½ pounds. However, just like the fitness walker, the fitness runner or fitness cyclist would improve only his or her cardiovascular fitness, not his or her muscular strength. Therefore, this high-intensity aerobic exerciser would still lose the same half pound of muscle with each birthday after age 35. And, of course, the high-intensity aerobic exerciser would still gain the same 2 pounds of fat by the end of the year. If you're over age 35 you would lose only about 13½ pounds in one year despite your 90 minutes per week intense running or cycling program.

3) Gold Coast Resistance Circuit-Training Workout

The 150-pound adult who performs our resistance circuit-training workout for 30 minutes three times a week would burn a total of 720 calories by the end of the week.

If you burn an additional 720 calories a week you can expect to lose 11 pounds in one year. But that's not the end of the story. Remember, instead of merely conditioning your cardiovascular system, our Gold Coast workout simultaneously builds lean muscle and therefore increases your resting metabolic rate. Increasing your resting metabolic rate is the key to attaining a lean, fit body in the shortest time possible.

It's difficult to say exactly how much muscle you'll gain on any resistance training program; there are numerous variables to take into consideration. Genetics, age and gender aside, with resistance training you have some control over the results you achieve. In other words: How muscular do you want to be? What are your personal aesthetic fitness goals? To get bigger muscles you simply choose to lift heavier weights. Once you are satisfied with your muscle mass, you can stop increasing the weight and focus on maintenance.

For the sake of simplicity, let's say the average unconditioned person who follows our Gold Coast Cure fitness program gains 4 pounds of muscle in the first few months of training. This is not at all unreasonable if you start out as an untrained individual. Four pounds of muscle burn 160 extra calories per day. This 160 extra calories burned every day results in a weight loss of 16½ pounds in one year.

At the end of the year, 11 pounds of fat are burned by the actual exercise. Four pounds of muscle are gained from the weight training, and 16½ pounds of fat are lost due to the increase in your metabolism from this muscle gain. Your total weight loss at the end of the year would be 23½ pounds.

Myth #3: If I'm not overweight, there is no need to perform resistance exercise.

Even if you're not overweight, you still lose metabolically active muscle with every birthday after about your thirty-fifth unless you perform some sort of resistance exercise. Again, each pound of muscle burns roughly 40 calories a day. Unless you strength train, you can expect to lose about a half pound of metabolically active muscle with each birthday from about age 35 on.

Getting Started

The Gold Coast Cure workout takes advantage of scientifically proven shortcuts to shape you up fast. We will show you how to get fit by doing less than 2 hours per week of total exercise. Resistance circuit-training is the secret.

The Gold Coast Cure workout challenges your muscles to grow stronger and challenges your heart to beat more efficiently. The Cure's resistance circuit-training workout routine includes aerobic-toning intervals plus strength training segments that burn mega-calories, build muscle and condition your cardiovascular system. Aerobic toning segments combine muscle-shaping exercises with cardiovascular conditioning in order to increase your lean body mass and blast fat fast. The routine strengthens and tones every major muscle group in your body. And because you won't be resting during your workout sessions, the routine burns a lot more calories in a lot less time than traditional weight training workouts that incorporate long rest periods between exercises.

Our workout turns untrained bodies into healthy, fit, fat-burning machines in the least amount of time possible. The workout takes a mere 30 minutes to complete, and each workout is performed only three times per week. For best results we suggest you perform our 10-minute core training routine twice a week also.

Adding Additional Aerobic Exercise

Though not required, performing extra aerobic exercise in addition to our Gold Coast workout will definitely speed your weight loss and increase your cardiovascular fitness level. We tend to recommend low-impact aerobics for this purpose. Good low-impact choices include fitness walking, swimming, cycling, elliptical machine training and step-aerobics.

Please understand we are absolutely *not* against aerobic exercise. However, if you're only going to exercise for a limited amount of time, resistance circuit-training is your best bet overall. If you're willing to exercise for more than two hours per week, then definitely add some aerobic exercise into the mix. Overweight individuals who incorporate extra aerobic exercise lose weight even faster than if they just do circuit-training exercise.

If super-speedy weight loss is your goal, try adding at least 20 minutes of aerobic exercise to our Gold Coast exercise program 2 or 3 days per week. To be sure you're giving it your all every time you exercise, it's best to perform purely aerobic exercise on the days you are not doing our resistance circuit-training workout.

Once you lose your excess weight you can stop doing the extra aerobics, but you must continue on with our workout if you want to keep your metabolic rate up and keep the weight off for good. Resistance exercise must become a permanent part of your new lifestyle if you want to enjoy Gold Coast health.

The 30-Minute Full-Body DVD Workout

The 30-minute workout on the accompanying DVD is slightly more challenging than the workout we provide in this book. If you are a beginner, you may want to start with the exercises in the book and work your way up to the DVD. You can also use the DVD workout— or any of the following routines—using no weights or lighter weights, and resting when you get tired.

It's good to vary the intensity of your workout to challenge your body and prevent boredom. You can mix and match your workouts, just be sure to give your muscles one day of rest between resistance workouts. Perform 30 minutes of resistance training 3 times a week.

Gold Coast Fitness Routine

This routine is designed for all fitness levels. If you are new to exercise, perform the repetitions suggested for Level 1 and use the lightest weights recommended. Beginner exercisers who are over the age of fifty may want to consider performing the workout several times without any weight. Experienced exercisers should increase the intensity and move to Level 2 while also increasing the amount of weight lifted. Increase the resistance slowly by adding two, three or five pounds to one or two exercises at a time.

This workout burns calories, blasts fat and builds muscle in just thirty minutes. You will condition your heart, lungs and every major muscle group in your body while you simultaneously improve muscle tone and increase your endurance. For best results, perform this workout three times a week on nonconsecutive days.

Equipment Needed

- *Cardio Equipment:*

  Level 1: A recumbent bicycle or a 4- to 8-inch tall step-up bench or 1-pound dumbbells.

  Level 2: A recumbent bicycle or a jump rope.

- *Step-Up Bench:*

  Level 1: 4- to 8-inch tall step-up bench, or use a single step in your house.

  Level 2: 10- to 12-inch step-up bench, or use two stairs in your house.

• *Dumbbells:*

Women:	Men:
Level 1 use 1, 3 and 5 pounds.	**Level 1** use 3, 5, and 7 pounds.
Level 2 use 3, 5 and 7 pounds.	**Level 2** use 5, 7, 10 and 15 pounds.

• A hand towel.
• A sturdy chair.
• A padded mat.
• A stopwatch is handy to guide your workout. You can wear this around your neck or on your wrist.

Training Tips

• When the directions say to perform an exercise "super slow," count to six while lifting the weight, then count to six again while lowering the weight.
• When the directions say to perform an exercise at a "moderate tempo," count to three while lifting the weight, then count to three again while lowering the weight.
• When doing any compound exercise that works your upper body and your lower body simultaneously, be sure to keep your abdominal muscles tight, your back straight and your shoulders back. Never curve your spine and shoulders forward, or you risk serious injury to your back.
• Focus on doing each exercise correctly with proper form.
• Don't get frustrated if at first the exercises seem confusing or awkward. Keep practicing. Soon you will memorize the routine and it will seem like second nature.
• Do not rest between exercises. Move from one exercise to the next without stopping. The first several times you try this workout, it will probably take you longer than 30 minutes to complete. Once you learn the routine, the entire workout takes no more than 30 minutes.

1. **Standing Alternating Knee Lifts.** Lift each knee 25 times for a *total* of 50 knee lifts. You should perform this exercise briskly.

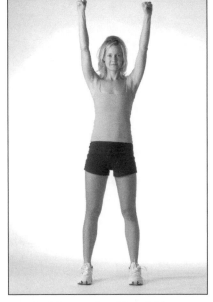 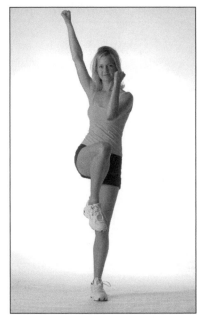

Stand with your feet hip-width apart and your arms held overhead.

Briskly bring your left elbow downward and your right knee upward. Your elbow and knee should meet at waist level. Return to standing position, then switch sides. Alternate knees for a total of 50 knee lifts.

2. 1-Minute Cardio Interval.

Level 1: Ride the recumbent bicycle at a high intensity, or do alternating high knee-raises while stepping up and down on your step-up bench, or vigorously march in place while holding 1-pound dumbbells.

Level 2: Ride the recumbent bicycle at a high intensity, jump rope or do jumping jacks.

3. Push-ups.

Level 1: Modified Push-ups. 12 reps. (Level 2 see next page)

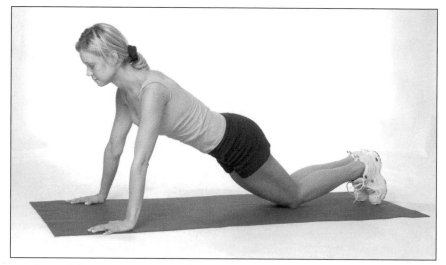

Kneel on all fours with your palms flat on the ground and shoulder-width apart. Keep your head, neck, spine and hips in a straight line. Contract your abdominal muscles.

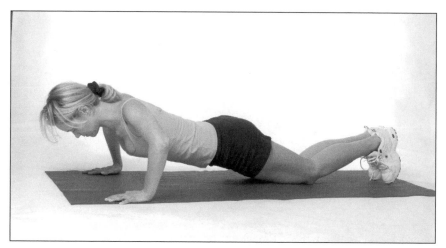

Slowly bend your elbows and lower your body down. Hold this position for a count of 2. Slowly push back up, then repeat.

Level 2: Full Push-up. 15–20 reps.

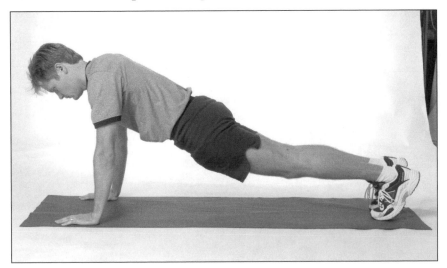

Place your hands shoulder-width apart with your fingers pointing forward. Keep your legs and torso straight.

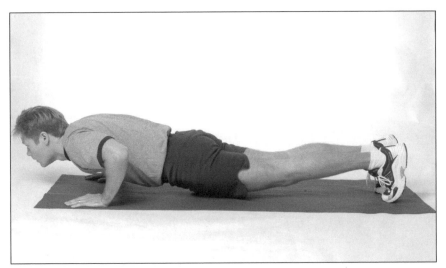

Slowly bend your elbows and lower your body down. Slowly push yourself back up to the start position and repeat.

4. Squats with Alternating Straight Side Leg Lifts.

Level 1: 18 reps. 9 lifts per leg.

Level 2: 22 reps. 11 lifts per leg.

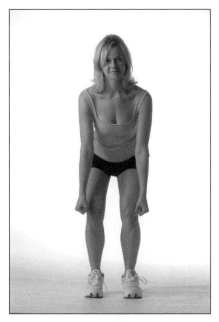 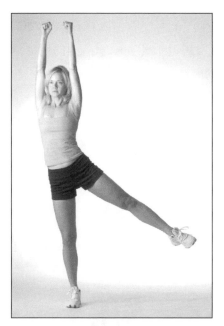

Squat with your feet hip-width apart and your knees bent at a 90-degree angle. Keep your arms straight down at your sides.

Stand up and extend a straightened LEFT leg out to the side while simultaneously raising both arms overhead. Lower your LEFT leg and arms as you squat back down into the start position. Repeat the movement, alternating legs.

5. Overhead Press.

MEN:	WOMEN:
Level 1 use 5 to 7 pounds.	**Level 1** use 3 to 5 pounds.
Level 2 use 10 to 15 pounds.	**Level 2** use 7 pounds.

Level 1: 4 reps super-slow + 8 reps at a moderate tempo (12 total reps).

Level 2: 6 reps super-slow + 8 reps at a moderate tempo (14 total reps).

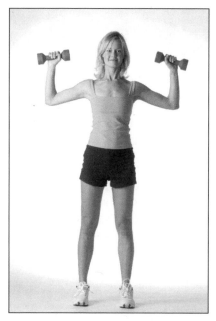 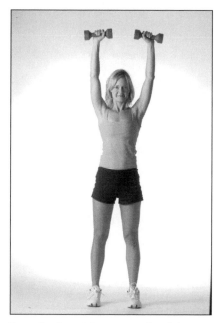

Stand with your feet hip-width apart. Hold a weight in each hand with your elbows bent and slightly below shoulder level. Palms should face forward.

Press both weights upward, raising your arms above your head; be careful not to lock your arms straight. Slowly lower the weights to the start position. Repeat.

6. Squats with Bicep Curls.

MEN:	WOMEN:
Level 1 use 5 to 7 pounds.	**Level 1** use 3 to 5 pounds.
Level 2 use 10 to 15 pounds.	**Level 2** use 7 pounds.

Level 1: 6 reps super slow + 6 reps at a moderate tempo (12 total reps).

Level 2: 8 reps super slow + 8 reps at a moderate tempo (16 total reps).

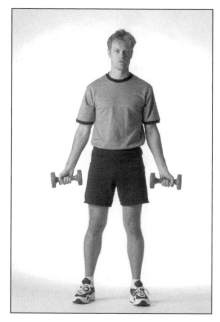 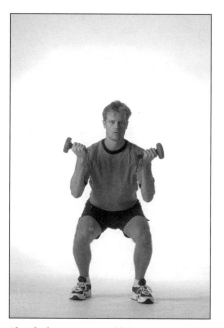

Stand with your feet hip-width apart. Hold your weights down at your sides with your elbows slightly bent, your palms should face forward.

Slowly lower yourself into a squatting position by bending your knees 90 degrees. Simultaneously bend your elbows and curl the weights toward your chest. As you stand back up, lower the weights back to hip-height. Repeat.

7. Standing Oblique Exercise.

Level 1: 20 reps. Each time one elbow touches one knee counts as 1 rep.

Level 2: 30 reps. Each time one elbow touches one knee counts as 1 rep.

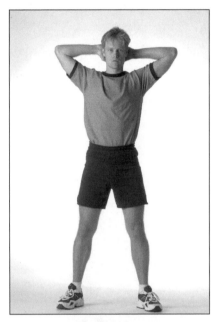 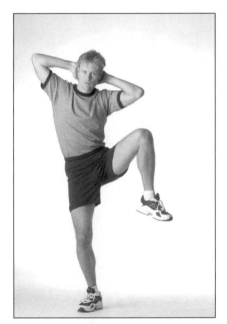

Stand with your feet hip-width apart and both of your hands clasped behind your head. Your elbows should be sticking out level with your ears.

Slowly lift your left knee up and out to the side while simultaneously bending your waist and lowering your left elbow to touch your knee. *Alternate* sides for the recommended number of reps.

8. 1-Minute Cardio Interval.

Level 1: Ride the recumbent bicycle at a high intensity, or do alternating high knee-raises while stepping up and down on your step-up bench, or vigorously march in place while holding 1-pound dumbbells.

Level 2: Ride the recumbent bicycle at a high intensity, jump rope or do jumping jacks.

9. Single-Leg Reverse Lunges off a Step-up Bench (or stairs).

MEN:

Level 1 use 3 to 5 pounds and a 4- to 8-inch-tall step-up bench or a single step in your house.

Level 2 use 7 pounds and a tall 10- to 12-inch step-up bench or 2 stairs in your house.

Level 1: 12 reps with each leg.

WOMEN:

Level 1 use 1 to 3 pounds and a 4- to 8-inch-tall step-up bench or a single step in your house.

Level 2 use 5 pounds and a tall 10- to 12-inch step-up bench or 2 stairs in your house.

Level 2: 15 reps with each leg.

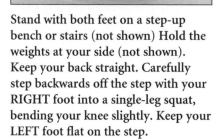 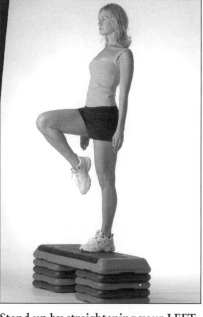

Stand with both feet on a step-up bench or stairs (not shown) Hold the weights at your side (not shown). Keep your back straight. Carefully step backwards off the step with your RIGHT foot into a single-leg squat, bending your knee slightly. Keep your LEFT foot flat on the step.

Stand up by straightening your LEFT leg and driving your RIGHT knee up towards your chest. Return to the start position and repeat the exercise for the recommended number of reps. Switch sides.

10. **"Towel Resistance" Bicep Curls.** Use a medium-sized hand towel.
   Level 1: 10 reps.
   Level 2: 12 reps.

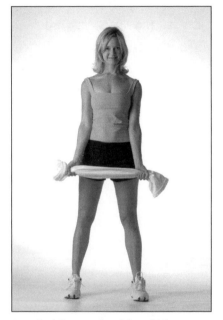 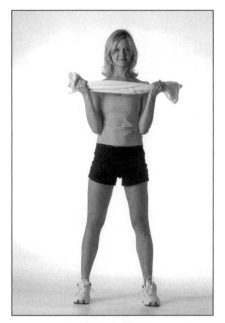

Stand with your feet hip-width apart. Hold a hand towel with both hands down in front of your hips and your palms facing forward. Do not bend your wrists. Pull against the towel evenly on both sides as if you were trying to pull it apart.

Continue trying to pull the towel apart while slowly curling the towel up towards your chest. Make sure to keep your elbows in close to your body and your shoulders motionless. Slowly lower the towel and repeat. *The harder you pull the more difficult this exercise will be.*

11. 1-Minute Cardio Interval.

Level 1: Ride the recumbent bicycle at a high intensity, or do alternating high knee-raises while stepping up and down on your step-up bench, or vigorously march in place while holding 1 pound dumbbells.

Level 2: Ride the recumbent bicycle at a high intensity, jump rope or do jumping jacks.

12. Forward Lunge.

MEN:	WOMEN:
Level 1 use 3 to 5 pounds.	**Level 1** use 1 to 3 pounds.
Level 2 use 7 to 10 pounds.	**Level 2** use 5 to 7 pounds.

Level 1: 10 reps with each leg.   **Level 2:** 12 reps with each leg.

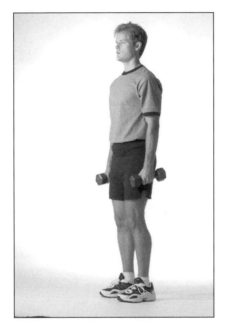

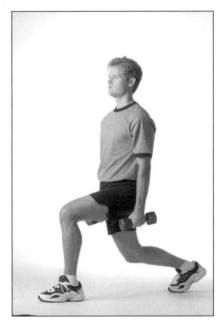

Stand with your feet shoulder-width apart and hold the dumbbells at your sides. Keep your back straight and abdominal muscles contracted.

Step forward about one stride-length from the back foot; make sure your knee does not extend beyond your toes. As you step forward, lower your body down and spring back to starting position, pushing through with the heel of your front foot. Repeat recommended number of reps and then switch sides.

13. 1-Minute Cardio Interval.

Level 1: Ride the recumbent bicycle at a high intensity, or do alternating high knee-raises while stepping up and down on your step-up bench, or vigorously march in place while holding 1-pound dumbbells.

Level 2: Ride the recumbent bicycle at a high intensity, jump rope or do jumping jacks.

14. Seated Super Slow Tricep Extensions.

MEN: WOMEN:

Level 1 use 5 to 7 pounds.   **Level 1** use 3 to 5 pounds.

Level 2 use 10 pounds.   **Level 2** use 7 pounds.

Level 1: 4 reps super slow + 8 reps at a moderate tempo (12 total reps).

Level 2: 4 reps super slow + 10 reps at a moderate tempo (14 total reps).

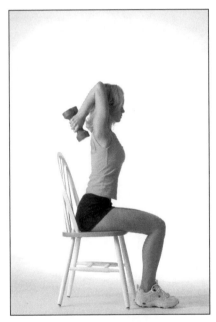   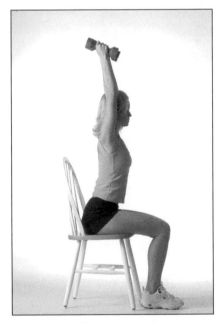

Sit on a chair while keeping your back straight and your abdominal muscles contracted. Clasp the dumbbells behind your head so that your elbows are level with your head.

Slowly extend your arms, keeping your elbows close together. Slowly return to the start position and repeat.

15. Plie with Chest Press.

MEN:	WOMEN:
Level 1 use 3 pounds.	**Level 1** use 1 pound.
Level 2 use 5 pounds.	**Level 2** use 3 pounds.
Level 1: 10 reps.	**Level 2:** 12 reps.

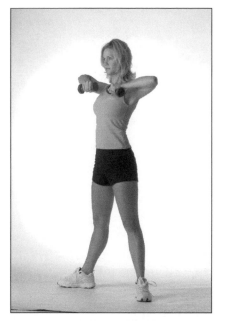 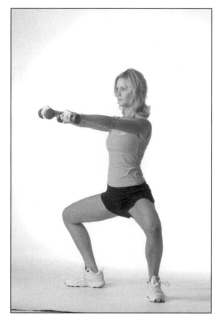

Stand with your feet shoulder-width apart and your toes turned out at a 45-degree angle. Contract your abdominal muscles while keeping your back straight. Hold a weight in each hand close to your body at chest level. Bend your elbows; your palms should be facing the floor.

Lower yourself down into a deep plie while straightening your elbows to push the weights out away from your body. Return your elbows to the starting position while simultaneously straightening your knees to stand back up. Repeat.

16. Squats and Squat Jumps.

Level 1: Squats with isometric contraction. 10 reps.

(Level 2 see next page.)

MEN use 7 pounds.   **WOMEN** use 5 pounds.

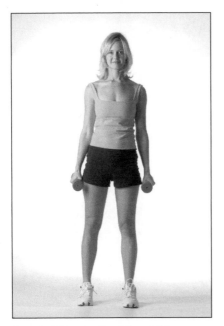

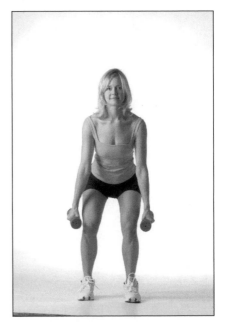

Stand with your feet hip-width apart, knees slightly bent. Keep your back straight and hold your weights at your sides.

Bend your knees to 90 degrees and allow your body to lean forward slightly; hold the squat position for a count of 6. Slowly return to the start position and repeat.

Level 2: Squat Jumps. 15 reps.

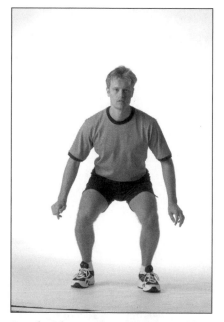 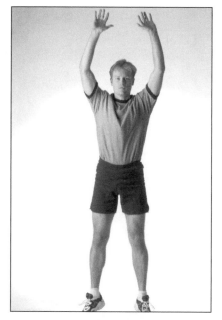

Stand with your feet shoulder width apart. Squat down slightly while keeping your chest lifted, your abdominal muscles contracted, and your shoulders back. Hold your arms straight down at your sides.

Use your glutes and thighs to jump up into the air while simultaneously thrusting your arms up toward the ceiling. You don't need to jump as high as possible. This exercise is very effective even if you only jump an inch or so. Land on your heels then roll forward onto your toes. Repeat.

17. One-Arm Dumbbell Row.

MEN:	WOMEN:
Level 1 use 7 pounds.	**Level 1** use 5 pounds.
Level 2 use 10 to 15 pounds.	**Level 2** use 7 pounds.

Level 1: 6 reps super slow + 6 reps at a moderate tempo (12 total reps).

Level 2: 6 reps super slow + 8 reps at a moderate tempo (14 total reps).

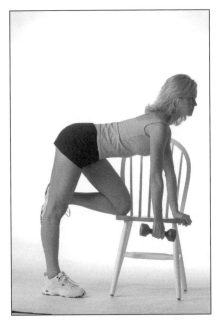 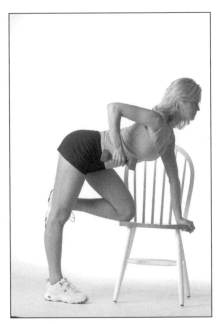

Straddle a sturdy chair with your left knee resting on the chair and your right foot flat on the floor. Bend forward at your waist to rest your left hand on the chair in front of your knee for support. Hold the weight in your right hand with your arm hanging at your side and your right palm facing in toward your body and the chair. Contract your abdominal muscles. Keep your back as straight and flat as possible.

Slowly bring your right elbow up toward the ceiling and back slightly toward your hip. Keep your elbow close to your body at all times. Slowly lower the weight down toward the ground as you bring it back to the start position. Repeat for the recommended number of reps and then switch sides.

18. Plie Squat with Upright Row.

MEN:	WOMEN:
Level 1 use 5 to 7 pounds.	**Level 1** use 3 to 5 pounds.
Level 2 use 10 to 15 pounds.	**Level 2** use 7 pounds.

Level 1: 6 reps super slow + 6 reps at a moderate tempo (12 reps total).

Level 2: 6 reps super slow + 8 reps at a moderate tempo (14 reps total).

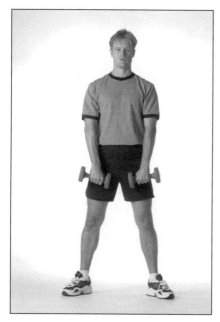 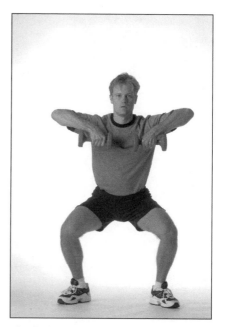

Stand with your feet shoulder-width apart and your toes turned out at a 45-degree angle. Contract your abdominal muscles while keeping your back straight. Hold the weights down in front of you with your palms facing towards your body.

Slowly bend your knees to lower your body to the ground while simultaneously pulling both weights up to chest level. Hold this position briefly. Slowly lower the weights back down as you straighten your legs back to a standing position. Repeat.

19. 1-Minute Alternating High Knee Raises with Alternating Arm Lifts.

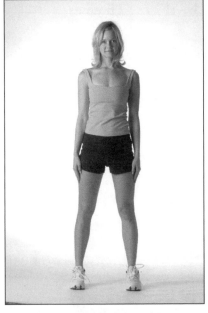 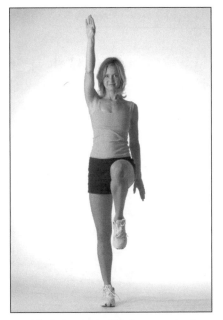

Stand with your feet hip-width apart and your arms down at your sides. Contract your abdominal muscles.

Briskly bring your left knee up in front of your chest and lift your right arm straight up in the air. Keep alternating sides for 1 minute. Move briskly and lift your knees as high as possible.

20. **Yoga Warrior I Pose.**

Level 1: Hold the pose while counting to 25. Switch sides. Repeat.

Level 2: Hold the pose while counting to 35. Switch sides. Repeat.

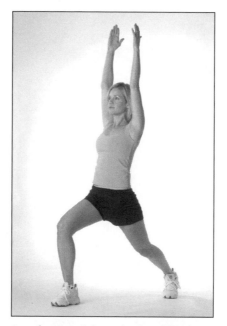

Stand up straight and take a large step back with your left foot, keeping hips and toes pointing forward. Your right knee should be bent and your left leg should be straight. Extend both arms straight up in the air, palms facing in. Hold the pose for 25–35 seconds, then switch sides.

21. 1-Minute Cardio Boxing with Squats.

MEN:	WOMEN:
Level 1 use 3 pounds.	**Level 1** use 1 pound.
Level 2 use 5 pounds.	**Level 2** use 3 pounds.

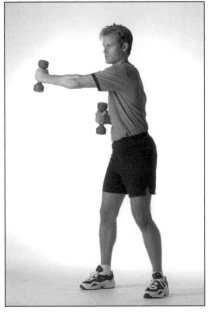 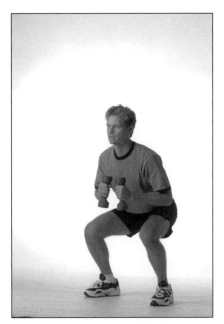

Stand with your feet hip-width apart and your abdominal muscles contracted. Hold the weights in your hands at chest level with your palms facing your chest and your elbows bent (not shown). In a controlled manner punch your left arm across your body, then bring it back to starting position. Never fully straighten your elbow when executing punches. Alternate punches left to right 6 times, 3 on each side.

Then do one squat: bend your knees to 90 degrees and allow your body to lean forward slightly. During your squat, hold the weights at chest level without punching. Repeat the sequence; 6 punches and 1 squat for a total of 1 minute.

22. Bent-over Lateral Raises.

MEN:	WOMEN:
Level 1 use 5 to 7 pounds.	**Level 1** use 3 pounds.
Level 2 use 10 pounds.	**Level 2** use 5 pounds.

Level 1: 4 reps super slow + 6 reps at a moderate tempo (10 total reps).

Level 2: 4 reps super slow + 8 reps at a moderate tempo (12 total reps).

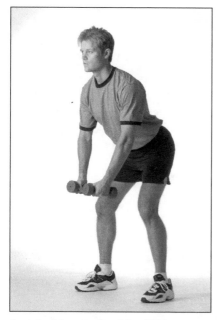 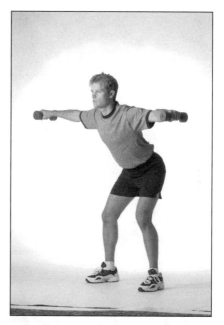

Stand with your feet hip-width apart, keeping your knees slightly bent. Bend forward very slightly, holding the weights in front of your hips and below your chest. Your palms should face each other and your elbows should be relaxed. Keep your head in line with your spine.

Raise your arms *out* to the side, lifting the weights until they are level with your shoulders. Return to the start position and repeat.

22. Repeat exercise #3 (Push-ups).

23. Kneeling Donkey Kicks.

   Level 1: 12 reps super slow.

   Level 2: 16 reps super slow.

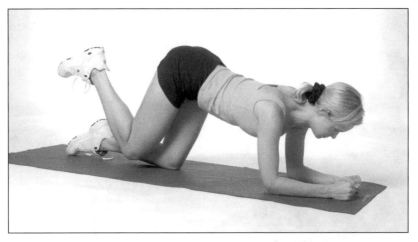

Support yourself on your elbows and left knee; lift your right knee slightly off the ground. Be sure to keep your back straight and abdominal muscles contracted.

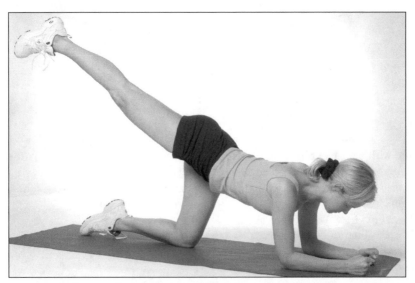

Slowly straighten and extend your right leg behind you. Hold your leg at the top for 2 seconds, then slowly lower it back down. Repeat all reps on your right leg and then switch sides.

24. Repeat exercise #4 (Squats with Alternating Straight Side Leg Lifts).

25. Upright rows.

MEN:	WOMEN:
Level 1 use 7 pounds.	**Level 1** use 5 pounds.
Level 2 use 10 to 15 pounds	**Level 2** use 7 pounds

Level 1: 6 reps super slow + 6 reps at a moderate tempo (12 total reps).

Level 2: 6 reps super slow + 8 reps at a moderate tempo (14 total reps).

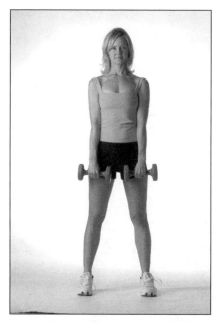

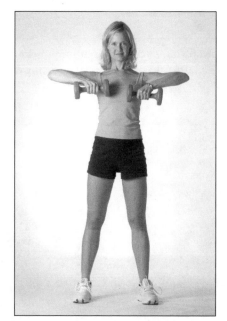

Stand with your feet hip-width apart, knees slightly bent and back straight. Hold the weights in front of you so that your palms face your thighs.

Pull the weights up to chest height, leading with the elbows. Slowly lower the weights and return to the start position. Repeat.

26. **Body Raise.**

Level 1: 15 reps super slow.

Level 2: 20 reps super slow.

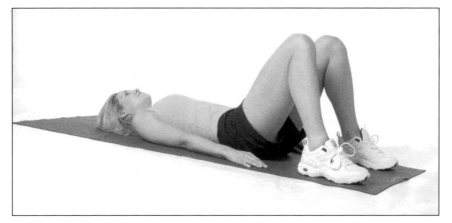

Lie on your back with your knees bent and your heels flat on the floor. Place your arms at your sides, palms facing down.

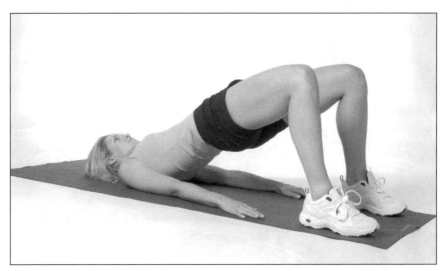

Slowly lift your pelvis and lower-back up off the floor. Squeeze your glutes and hold the position for 2 seconds and then slowly lower yourself back down to the start position. Repeat.

Congratulations! You've completed the workout. You should perform this routine three times weekly. Do not attempt this workout on back-to-back days. Give your muscles time to rest between workouts.

Don't forget to supplement this workout with our ten-minute core training workout two times per week. You can either do your core training at the end of this workout or on a separate day. If you want to do more exercise than this, try some form of low-impact aerobic exercise such as walking, swimming or biking one, two or three times a week.

10-Minute Core Training Workout

The core training exercises are designed to be done twice weekly. Our entire core training routine can be completed in only 10 minutes. You can either do your core training workout on the same day as your 30-minute resistance-circuit training workout or on alternate days. The only equipment required is a padded mat and light dumbbells weighing 3, 5 or 7 pounds. Although the core training workout is essentially the same for all fitness levels, beginners should perform these exercises at level 1 while more advanced exercises should perform these exercises at level 2.

It is important to perform all of the core training exercises slowly and steadily. The more slowly and intensely you focus on each position, the better your results will be. Pay close attention to directions instructing you to hold a given position. When you hold a position at peak contraction, you maximize recruitment of the muscle fibers being worked and you dramatically intensify the exercise.

1. Swan Sweep.

Level 1: Perform 6 to 8 reps.

Level 2: Perform 10 to 12 reps.

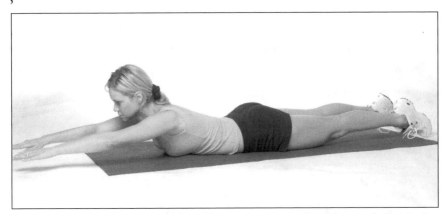

Lie on your stomach with your chest down. Your arms should extend straight in front of you and your palms should face the floor. Slightly lift your shoulders, arms, head and chest off the ground while pressing your hips, legs and feet into the ground.

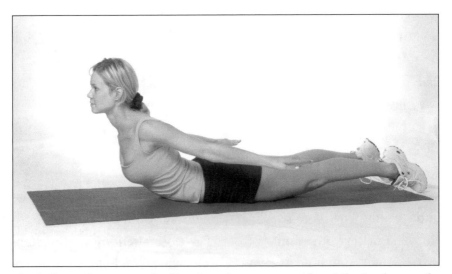

Slowly "sweep" your arms backwards and out to your sides while simultaneously lifting your shoulders higher off the ground. Keep your arms straight. Your elbows should bend minimally. Once your arms have gone back as far as they can comfortably go, return to the start position. Repeat.

2. **Opposite Arm, Opposite Leg.**

Level 1: Perform 8 super slow reps on each side.

Level 2: Perform 10 super slow reps on each side.

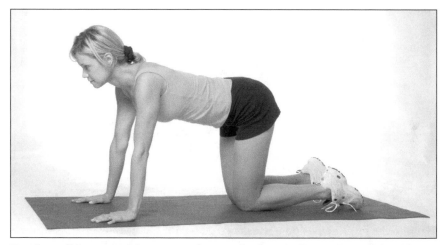

Kneel on all fours. Position your palms on the floor in line with your shoulders and your knees on the floor in line with your hips. Contract your abdominal muscles so your back forms a straight line from your head to your hips.

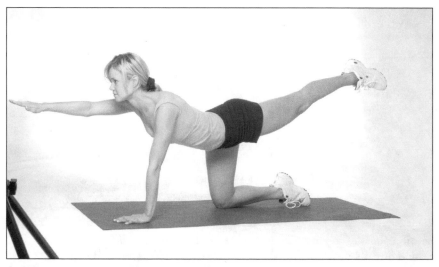

Stabilize your spine and keep your abdominal muscles contracted. Slowly and carefully lift your right arm in front of you and your left leg straight out behind you to hip height. Hold this position for a count of 2. Lower and repeat. Complete *all* the reps on one side, then switch sides.

3. Yoga Plank Pose.

Level 1: Hold this pose for 60 counts. (Level 2 see below.)

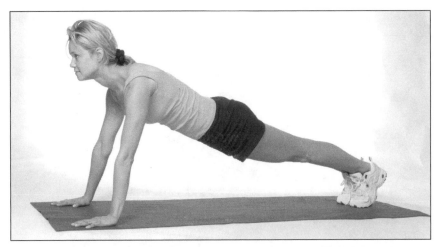

Get into the push-up position by balancing on your toes with your arms straight and your palms on the ground directly under your shoulders. Keep your body straight and your head in alignment with your spine. Contract your abdominal muscles and squeeze your butt and inner thighs together as tight as possible. Hold this position for 60 counts.

Level 2: Hold this pose for 60 counts.

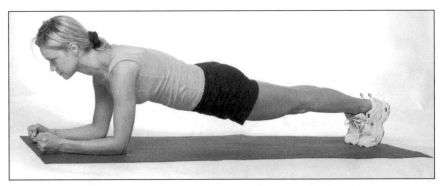

Position yourself so your toes are on the ground and your *elbows* are on the ground directly beneath your shoulders. Carefully raise your body up while keeping a straight line from your shoulders to your ankles. Support the weight of your body by balancing on your forearms and your toes. Contract your abdominal muscles and squeeze your butt and inner thighs together. Hold the position for 60 counts.

4. Hamstring Stretch.

Level 1 and Level 2: Hold the stretch for 20 seconds, switch legs, then repeat.

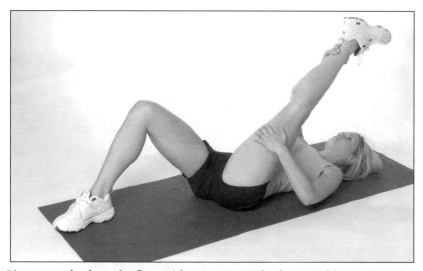

Lie on your back on the floor with your RIGHT leg bent. Hold your LEFT leg with one hand behind your thigh and one hand behind your calf muscle. Keeping your LEFT leg as straight as possible, gently pull it toward you until you feel slight tension down the back of your leg. Hold the position for a count of 20. Switch sides.

5. **Weighted Abdominal Crunch.**

Level 1: 12 reps, 3 pounds.

Level 2: 15 reps, 5 or 7 pounds.

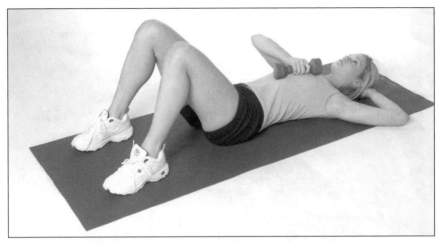

Lie on your back with your feet flat on the floor and your knees bent. Place your left hand behind your head. Hold the weight in your right hand and place the weight gently on your chest. Keep both elbows out to the side. Focus your eyes on the ceiling. *Keep your chin off your chest. Imagine you are holding an apple under your chin.*

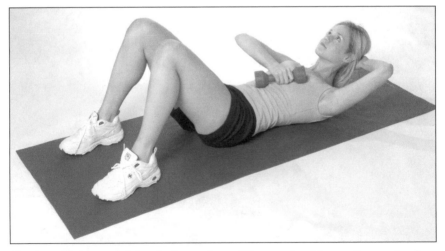

Slowly contract your abdominal muscles to lift your shoulders and upper back forward a few inches off the ground. *Remember, don't bend your chin forward keep the apple in place!* Hold the position for 2 seconds, then slowly return to the start position.

6. **Oblique Crunch.**

Level 1: 8 reps each side.

Level 2: 12 reps each side.

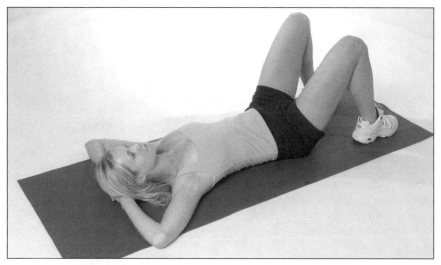

Lie on your back with your feet flat on the floor and your knees bent. Place both hands behind your head with both elbows out to your side.

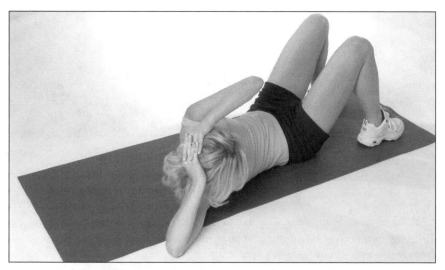

Contract your abdominal muscles. Slowly lift your head, neck and shoulders off the ground. Rotate your left elbow toward your right knee. *Hold the position for 5 seconds.* Slowly return to the start position. Do *all* of the reps on one side before switching sides.

7. Inner Thigh Beats.

Level 1: Count to 30.

Level 2: Count to 60.

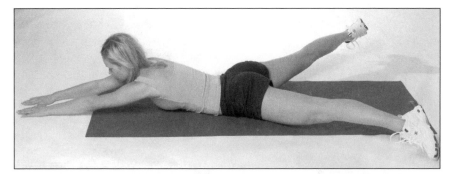

Lie on your stomach with your arms straight out in front of you. Keep your legs behind you slightly more than *hip-width* apart. Contract your abdominal muscles and press your pelvic bones into the ground, then lift both of your legs up a couple inches off the ground.

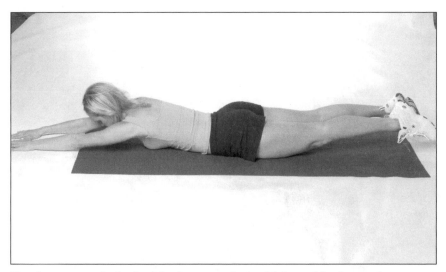

Keeping your entire body tight, beat your inner thighs and heels together. Repeat this in-and-out motion as you count out the reps.

8. Yoga Airplane Pose.

Level One: Count to 30 on each side.
Level Two: Count to 40 on each side.

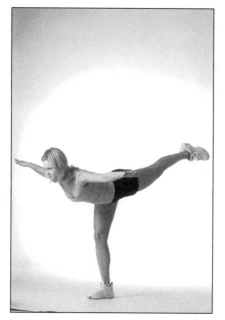

Step forward on your right foot with your right knee slightly bent. Find your balance. Bend forward from your hips, pushing your left leg behind you. Lift your left leg off the ground and lean your body forward. Your torso and your left leg should end up parallel to the ground while you stand on your right foot *only.* Now extend both arms straight out to the side like airplane wings. Hold the position. *Beginners may need to hold on to a chair with one hand for support.* Switch sides and repeat.

9. Standing Tick Tocks.

   Level One: 16 reps.

   Level Two: 20 reps.

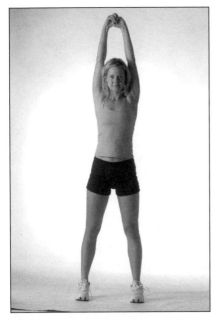 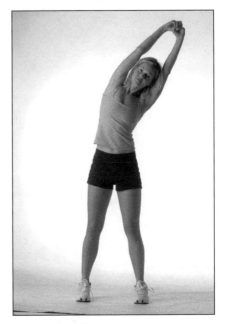

Stand with your feet slightly shoulder-width apart. Clasp your hands and hold your arms straight overhead.

Tuck your pelvis and contract your abdominal muscles. Slowly bend to the left at your waist as far as you can comfortably go. Return to the start position. Alternate sides until you complete the desired number of reps.

Supplements Made Simple: Your Daily Vitamin Planner

11

Optimal health is not the mere absence of disease; it's being in peak mental and physical shape while having the energy and vitality to live life to the fullest.

You can achieve approximately 90 percent of optimal health through a combination of proper nutrition, appropriate exercise, proper sleep and effective stress management. However, modern science can take you one step further. Research shows that certain vitamins and minerals, taken in supplement form at doses greater than the minimum amount required to avoid disease, provide health benefits above and beyond what can be achieved with diet and exercise alone. In fact, many of the best medical doctors routinely include nutritional supplements as part of their treatment plan for certain diseases, sometimes in conjunction with prescription medication, and sometimes as the primary treatment. The Gold Coast Cure discusses only those relatively few vitamin, mineral and nutritional supplements medically proven to help you live longer and live better.

The vitamins and supplements we discuss are designed to work in combination with our dietary and exercise advice. No pill can substitute for good nutrition, and you can't find the benefits of exercise in any bottle. This having been said, it is our belief, and the belief of esteemed organizations such as the American Medical Association, that select vitamins, minerals and essential fat supplements complement even the most healthful diet.

Surely you've seen vitamin content expressed in percentage terms on the labeling of the packaged food products you purchase. These reference daily intakes (RDIs) for vitamins and minerals are adequate for maintaining life and adequate for preventing rare diseases caused by severe vitamin deficiency. These RDIs are not necessarily adequate for attaining optimal health.

Young, healthy adults who eat nutrient-rich, balanced diets can remain almost optimally healthy whether or not they consume supplemental amounts of the vitamins and minerals we recommend. These people are in the minority. Any individual who fits into any one of the categories we list in Table 11.1 will benefit from supplementation. Many of you will find that you fit into several of these categories. You have significantly increased nutritional needs, and this chapter is of special importance to you.

Table 11.1 People Who Significantly Benefit from Supplementation

Men over 35
Women over 45
Growing children and growing teenagers
Pregnant women and women trying to become pregnant
Nursing mothers
Cardiac patients
Competitive athletes
Persons under severe mental or physical stress
Burn victims
Anyone with an active infection
Heavy drinkers and recovering alcoholics
Anyone recovering from surgery
Diabetics
Asthmatics
People suffering from autoimmune diseases

Many prescription drugs increase your vitamin requirements substantially. The drugs most often implicated include antibiotics, chemotherapeutic agents, drugs used to prevent pregnancy and seizures, and drugs used to treat inflammatory conditions. Steroid drugs such as prednisone are particularly likely to increase vitamin requirements. A detailed discussion of this subject is beyond the scope of this book. We encourage you to read up on or ask your doctor about any prescription drugs you take. Always make sure your overall health is not compromised in a misguided attempt to treat an isolated symptom.

It's also important to remember that dietary supplementation of any type does not offer an overnight "cure" for any condition. The benefits from nutritional supplementation occur only after long-term commitment and long-term use. Consistency is crucial.

Vitamins, minerals and supplements can help you win your battle with the bulge. Many nutritionists blame our obesity epidemic, in part, on malnutrition. We've already discussed this connection in chapter 1. Blaming obesity on malnutrition may seem contradictory, but remember that malnutrition has nothing to do with how many calories you eat. Malnutrition means not getting the nutrients your body needs. If you overnourish yourself with nutrient-poor foods, you'll find yourself overweight but malnourished. In addition to contributing to food cravings, malnutrition interferes with your metabolism. You can't burn fat efficiently when the proper nutrients aren't in place to fuel fat-burning. If your body is properly nourished, it will have an internal monitor that regulates appetite, maintains a healthy body weight and burns fat. On the other hand, malnutrition slows your metabolism. Specifically, deficiencies of the essential fats, vitamin C and calcium may slow your metabolic rate substantially. A sluggish metabolism is a surefire way to get fat and stay that way.

The First Supplement You Need: Your Daily Multivitamin, Multimineral

Taking a multivitamin, multimineral supplement is the simplest, most important, least expensive way to improve your overall health. With one supplement you fill nutrient gaps, optimize your energy level, improve your brain function and help prevent disease.

In the past there was some controversy as to whether supplementation was really necessary. Today, we know for a fact that good-quality vitamin and mineral supplementation is an inexpensive health insurance policy and an inexpensive means to achieve improved quantity and quality of life.

In the *Journal of the American Medical Association,* it was recently recommended that all adults take a multivitamin every day.[1] Most of us are not eating enough nutrient-rich whole foods to meet even basic minimal vitamin and mineral requirements, and because certain vitamins and minerals in supplement form have been scientifically proven to reduce your risk of at least three highly prevalent degenerative conditions—cardiovascular disease, cancer and osteoporosis—it makes sense to supplement with a high-quality multivitamin.

Which multivitamin do you take? Good question, especially considering there are literally hundreds from which to choose. We suggest several high-quality brands beginning on page 264.

Do You Need Extra Folate?

Most multivitamin pills contain 400 micrograms of folate, equivalent to 100 percent of the RDI. Pregnant women, women trying to become pregnant and people with established cardiovascular disease (heart attack, stroke, claudication or dementia) should double or triple this dose. People with high homocysteine levels should also consider doubling or tripling the recommended folate dose. Unfortunately, obtaining this amount almost always requires taking a separate folate pill as it is very difficult to locate standard multivitamins containing more than 400 micrograms of folate. Consider discussing high-dose folate supplementation with your doctor.

The Second Supplement You Need: Calcium with Magnesium and Vitamin D

It's easy to find these three complementary nutrients together in one supplement. Let's discuss calcium first because the vast majority of us fail to meet minimum calcium requirements from diet alone.

While we all know that we need calcium to build strong bones, you may not be aware your bones need a *continuous* supply of calcium and other related bone-building nutrients throughout your lifetime in order to stay strong and healthy. Your bones are under perpetual construction; they are living organs that are constantly being broken down and rebuilt. They need a steady stream of bone-building "materials" to keep this process going.

Ideally, osteoporosis prevention should start before you reach age thirty-five. After about this age your bone density is already on the decline. If you are already older, don't be discouraged. No matter how old you happen to be, you should always think "prevention," as your bones are under constant reconstruction. Calcium supplementation has been proven in very high-quality studies to prevent bone loss in postmenopausal women.[2] It is never too late to start supplementing your diet with calcium.

Adults need between 1,000 milligrams and 1,200 milligrams of calcium every day. The National Institutes of Health claim the preferred way to get your calcium is through food. We agree. It has been argued your body absorbs as little as 30 percent of the calcium found in typical supplements. Consequently, in addition to supplementing with calcium you also need to eat the calcium-rich foods we discussed in chapter 3.

Calcium is good for fighting more than just osteoporosis. This mineral also helps prevent colon cancer.[3] "Waist watchers" may be especially interested in learning more about the connection between calcium and weight loss. According to research conducted at the University of Tennessee in Knoxville, high-calcium diets are very likely to reduce body fat stores based upon animal, epidemiological and clinical studies.[4] Michael Zemel, Ph.D., director of the Department of Nutrition at the university, explains, "Higher calcium diets favor burning fat rather than storing it." More recent research suggests, but does not prove, calcium *supplementation* may also help with weight loss.[5]

Vitamin D and magnesium are ideal partners for calcium because you need these two substances in significant concentrations in order to absorb and utilize calcium. If your body can't absorb and use the calcium supplements you take, you're wasting time and money. Furthermore, excess calcium intake, when combined with deficiencies of other equally essential bone-building nutrients, can actually cause your bones to become brittle and fragile and may even lead to clogged arteries.

Magnesium and vitamin D have highly beneficial effects of their own. Women who supplement with at least 400 international units (IUs) of vitamin D daily are more than one-third less likely to develop multiple sclerosis.[6] Magnesium is an effective antiarrhythmic drug that can stabilize your heartbeat. And magnesium supplementation can help decrease your blood pressure.[7] Again, your body needs a balance of nutrients in order to function optimally.

The ideal supplementation regimen provides a total of 1,000 milligrams of calcium, 400 milligrams of magnesium and 400 IUs of vitamin D per day. While to some people our recommended calcium dose may seem a little low, remember that most multivitamin, multimineral supplements also contain some calcium, some magnesium and even some vitamin D. Also, because the Gold Coast Cure diet is rich in natural nutrients, you'll obtain some of these bone-building nutrients from the whole foods you'll be eating. Excessive supplementation with calcium, magnesium and vitamin D is neither necessary nor healthful. See our Supplement Shopping Guide and our Daily Vitamin

Planner at the end of this chapter for brand-name suggestions and a sample supplementation schedule.

The Third Supplement You Need: Natural Vitamin E with Selenium

These two antioxidants are often found packaged together because they work synergistically. Vitamin E is an essential fat-soluble vitamin and a powerful antioxidant with numerous therapeutic properties. Unfortunately, no matter how perfect your diet may be, it is impossible to eat enough vitamin E–rich food to obtain maximal antioxidant benefit.

In synergy with various other antioxidants, vitamin E helps delay the effects of aging by preventing free radicals from damaging your cell membranes. Studies have shown vitamin E to be helpful in reducing blood pressure, decreasing the risk of stroke, inhibiting platelet aggregation, improving memory, reducing the overall number of deaths that occur due to heart disease and enhancing the immune system.

Vitamin E provides powerful protection against blood vessel disease by preventing cholesterol that is already in your bloodstream from oxidizing. Remember, cholesterol oxidation is partly responsible for the formation and growth of those artery-clogging plaque deposits that lead to cardiovascular disease. Vitamin E also inhibits platelet aggregation, providing additional protection against heart disease. Vitamin E and vitamin C, the next essential supplement on our list, work together to reduce your risk of Alzheimer's disease by more than 50 percent.[8]

It is important to take natural, as opposed to synthetic, vitamin E. Natural vitamin E delivers twice the antioxidant protection of synthetic vitamin E. Natural vitamin E is absorbed better from your digestive system and retained within your body longer. It's true that natural vitamin E is a bit more expensive than synthetic versions, but you get what you pay for. When shopping for vitamin E supplements, look at the ingredient list. You will see either "d-alpha" tocopherol, "dl-alpha" tocopherol or "mixed" tocopherols listed as the source of vitamin E. You want either the "d-alpha" tocopherol version or the "mixed" tocopherol version of vitamin E, *not* the synthetic "dl-alpha" version.

Be aware that vitamin E does thin the blood somewhat. If you are having surgery within the next week, or if you are already taking prescription-strength blood thinners such as aspirin, Plavix or Coumadin, it is worth talking about vitamin E supplementation with your family doctor, internist or cardiologist. In most cases we believe you should take vitamin E in addition to any prescription-strength blood thinners you might be taking, but every individual situation is different. Again, talk to your doctor first.

There has been increasing controversy of late about the health consequences of vitamin E supplementation. One recent study even suggests vitamin E supplementation may increase your risk of dying.[9] This study is intriguing, but there are weaknesses in its design. We have taken natural vitamin E for many years, and we believe there is enough evidence supporting the use of this antioxidant that we continue to do so.

Most of you will also choose to take the essential fat supplements, evening primrose oil and fish oil, that we recommend later. Vitamin E should be taken at the same time as any essential fat supplement you choose to take. Vitamin E prevents the oxidation of essential fats and helps maximize the potency of essential fat supplements. Without the antioxidant protection found in vitamin E, these essential fat supplements may partially oxidize after you ingest them, reducing their effectiveness significantly. Oxidized fats of *any* type can be harmful; many essential fat supplements contain a *little bit* of vitamin E for just this purpose. For best results follow our Daily Vitamin Planner near the end of this chapter.

Selenium

Now let's talk about selenium, vitamin E's best antioxidant mineral friend. These two substances work together to prevent free radical damage from accumulating inside your body. As a detoxifier, selenium helps escort toxins out of your system. This mineral is also vital for the production of your body's most plentiful self-made antioxidant, glutathione.

Research suggests selenium may provide protection against several forms of cancer, including lung cancer, prostate cancer and stomach cancer. One major Finnish study found that high blood levels of selenium significantly reduced the incidence of lung cancer in men.[10] Although adults need about 70 micrograms (100 percent of the RDI) of selenium per day for homeostasis, studies show maximal cancer prevention benefits occur when taking around 200 micrograms daily. As with every supplement we've discussed, don't overdo it. Consuming more than 400 micrograms per day of selenium may cause nerve damage, hair loss and brittle nails.

We suggest you take a brand containing 400 IU of natural vitamin E and between 100 micrograms and 200 micrograms of selenium. As we said earlier, these two antioxidants are often sold combined in one pill. This dose is in addition to any smaller amounts of vitamin E and selenium you might obtain from food and from your multivitamin, multimineral supplement. See our Supplement Shopping Guide and Daily Vitamin Planner at the end of this chapter for a list of brands to choose from and for suggestions as to when to take your vitamin E supplement.

The Fourth Supplement You Need: Vitamin C with Bioflavonoids

Vitamin C is a potent, extremely versatile antioxidant with roughly three hundred different functions in your body. For one, it helps mop up damaging free radicals before they have a chance to prematurely age your cells. Vitamin C also has the ability to regenerate other antioxidants, significantly boosting the overall antioxidant efficiency of your body. In combination with vitamin E supplementation, vitamin C supplementation has been proven to decrease the progression of artery disease.[11]

Diabetics often have low levels of vitamin C. This is because vitamin C is transported to the cells with the assistance of insulin, and diabetics are resistant to the actions of insulin. Diabetics often cannot distribute enough vitamin C to their cells even when they consume adequate amounts of this nutrient in their diets. It is therefore especially important for the diabetic to supplement with vitamin C.

And because vitamin C decreases histamine production, people who suffer from asthma may also find vitamin C supplements extremely helpful.

We suggest you take about 1,000 milligrams of supplemental vitamin C daily in addition to the amount that is contained in your multivitamin, multimineral pill. Your daily vitamin C regimen should also contain 200 milligrams to 500 milligrams of bioflavonoids as well. Bioflavonoids are essential for the absorption of vitamin C; they also enhance and boost the activity of vitamin C within your cells. You can easily find high-quality supplements containing vitamin C with bioflavonoids. See our Supplement Shopping Guide and Daily Vitamin Planner at the end of this chapter for a list of brands to choose from and suggestions as to exactly when to take these supplements.

Two Additional Nonvitamin Supplements You Need

That's it as far as the vitamins and minerals are concerned. But we're not done just yet. It's every bit as important to supplement with essential fats. Think of the essential fats as "vitamin fats."

Gamma Linolenic Acid (GLA)

GLA (gamma linolenic acid) is a special omega-6 fat that happens to be a direct building block for several *good* anti-inflammatory hormones. Because of this, GLA is the most helpful omega-6 fat from the standpoint of achieving optimal health. Unfortunately, GLA is *not* found in commonly eaten foods.

Whole foods rich in omega-6 fat such as sunflower seeds, sesame seeds and wheat germ contain an omega-6 fat called LA (linoleic acid). LA has the potential to be converted by your body into GLA, but this process can be thwarted by many internal and external factors. For example, the older you are, the less efficient the enzymes your body uses to convert LA into GLA. Chronic health conditions such as diabetes, malnutrition, infection and stress further reduce your body's ability to convert dietary LA into GLA.

Fortunately, supplementation with GLA is simple and affordable. GLA is naturally prevalent in the oils derived from four plant seeds: borage oil, evening primrose oil, hemp oil and black currant oil. Of these four oils, borage oil has the highest percent of GLA content. However, we recommend using evening primrose oil instead because this supplement has been more widely researched and it also seems to be the most easily available. It's important to choose a high-quality brand such as Barlean's Organic Evening Primrose Oil.

The Health Benefits of GLA

Supplementing with GLA can provide the following health benefits:

- Increase in your metabolic rate and enhanced weight loss.
- Dramatically reduced hormone-mediated nuisance symptoms. This means less severe premenstrual syndrome, decreased cyclical breast pain, less cramping, less bloating and less moodiness.
- Improved hair, nail, and skin health. Specifically, you will notice

thicker hair, stronger nails, less acne, and a reduced severity of inflammatory skin conditions such as eczema and psoriasis.

- Decreased tendency toward inflammation in general. This delivers benefits to people suffering from conditions such as fibromyalgia, asthma, multiple sclerosis, arthritis, Crohn's disease and so forth.
- Improvement in the symptoms of diabetic neuropathy.[12]
- Lowered bad LDL cholesterol and improved cholesterol ratio.[13]

How Much GLA Should You Take?

We recommend supplementing with 1,300 milligrams of evening primrose oil daily. However, if you already have an inflammation-mediated condition, you may benefit from taking up to two to three times as much GLA as we recommend. See our Daily Vitamin Planner near the end of this chapter for guidance as to when to take your GLA supplement.

Fish Oil with EPA and DHA

If you supplement with omega-6 GLA, you should also take an omega-3-rich fish oil supplement.

As discussed in chapter 6, EPA and DHA are the two omega-3 essential fats found in fish oil, and they are direct building blocks for several good anti-inflammatory hormones. Although we advocate eating fatty fishes such as salmon, herring, sea bass and sardines three to four times a week, you will obtain even better results with the assistance of omega-3 fat supplementation. If you refuse to eat fish for whatever reason, you *especially* need to supplement with the essential omega-3 fats found in fish oil supplements.

The benefits of supplementation with the EPA and DHA found in fish oil are numerous and include:

- Improved cholesterol profile
- Reversal of the metabolic syndrome

- Reduced risk of stroke, heart attack and congestive heart failure.
- Reduced risk of peripheral vascular disease.
- Better mental function, including an improved ability to concentrate and memorize.
- Reduced severity of Alzheimer's disease. Significantly reduced risk of developing dementia.

Choose only the highest-quality fish oil supplements you can find. Be sure the container used to package your fish oil supplement protects them completely from light and air. We recommend you take your fish oil supplement at the same time you take your vitamin E supplement.

A High-Quality Fish Oil Supplement

A brief word about our favorite fish oil supplement manufacturer, Nordic Naturals. This company guarantees their products have no "fishy" aftertaste. Nordic Naturals makes the freshest, purest fish oils we have yet to find. The oxidation level of fish oils is a key marker of freshness, and Nordic Naturals has been shown to have the lowest oxidation level of the top five brands. Nordic Naturals was also the only fish oil tested that was completely free of lead. Nordic Naturals products undergo rigid quality control procedures, including molecular distillation, and they surpass all national and international standards for environmental pollutants, including dioxins, PCBs, pesticides and heavy metals. Just remember that higher-quality supplements yield higher-quality results.

EPA and DHA work synergistically. These two fats must be supplemented together to produce optimal results. We recommend you supplement with at least 1,000 milligrams to 2,000 milligrams of combined EPA and DHA daily. If you refuse to eat fatty fish, we strongly suggest you take 2,000 milligrams of combined EPA and

DHA in supplement form daily in order to obtain an adequate amount of omega-3 essential fat.

Be aware that total essential fatty acid (essential fat) content is not equivalent to total EPA and DHA content. If the label boldly claims two pills contain "2,000 milligrams of omega-3 fatty acids," you are not necessarily getting 2,000 milligrams of combined EPA and DHA. Read the label carefully. Add up the total amount of EPA and DHA found in each serving. For example, if the front of the label reads "2,000 milligrams of omega-3 fatty acids" but the back side states one serving contains 360 milligrams of EPA and 240 milligrams of DHA, you are only getting 600 total milligrams of combined EPA and DHA. Be sure you get what you are paying for. Know exactly how many pills you have to take. In most cases, it's necessary to take at least two pills per day to obtain adequate amounts of omega-3 essential fat in supplement form.

Your Daily Vitamin Planner

It's important that some vitamins and supplements be taken together and some supplements be taken separately for maximal absorption. It's best to take all your supplements with food during the three main meals you eat each day. Be sure to follow the serving-size suggestions provided on the back of the supplement label because each brand varies slightly. For example, with some brands you need to take three capsules every day, and with some brands all the nutrients you need are found in just one pill. Some supplements, such as calcium and vitamin C, must be split into multiple doses because it's not possible to absorb all you need in one dose. Try to follow our daily vitamin planner as closely as possible.

Take at Breakfast

- Take the entire multivitamin, multimineral supplement.
- Take half your daily dose of vitamin C with bioflavonoids. Half your daily dose contains about 500 milligrams of vitamin C and about 100 to 250 milligrams of bioflavonoids.
- Take half your daily dose of calcium with magnesium and vitamin D. Half your daily dose contains about 500 milligrams of calcium, 200 milligrams of magnesium and 200 IU of vitamin D.

Take at Lunch

- Take the other half of your daily dose of vitamin C with bioflavonoids.
- Take the other half of your daily dose of calcium with magnesium and vitamin D.

Take at Dinner

- Take the entire daily dose of natural vitamin E with selenium. The daily dose contains about 400 IU of vitamin E and about 100 micrograms to 200 micrograms of selenium.
- Take the entire daily dose of GLA. We recommend you take about 1,300 milligrams of evening primrose oil so you get about 130 milligrams of GLA per day.
- Take the entire daily dose of fish oil containing both DHA and EPA. This daily dose should contain between 1,000 milligrams and 2,000 milligrams of combined EPA and DHA.

Note: Young people over the age of twelve can take the adult dosage of all of the recommended supplements. Specific recommendations for children twelve and under appear at the end of this chapter.

The Gold Coast Cure
Supplement Shopping Guide

All of the following supplements meet Gold Coast Cure standards for quality. All contain the vitamins and minerals your body needs in optimal doses. If you choose to take different brands, perhaps to save money, it's crucial you choose products of the highest quality that contain approximately the same dosages in approximately the same combination we have recommended in the text of this chapter. Doses do not need to be exactly the same, but they should be very close. Read labels carefully to determine how many pills or how many teaspoons are needed to make one serving.

We offer one more unsolicited comment. The Vitamin Shoppe is our favorite place to shop for these high-quality supplements. This store stocks high-quality products and offers significant discounts over retail prices. You may order many of these supplements online at *www.thevitaminshoppe.com.* You may also call 1-800-233-1216 for directions to a store near you.

Multivitamin, multimineral supplement

1. **Product made by:** Century Systems, Inc.
   Product name: Miracle 2000
   We recommend: One ounce (one capful), taken once a day
   Where to purchase: *www.thevitaminshoppe.com,* or just about any well-stocked vitamin store, or call the company direct at 1-800-The-Woman

   Note: This is a liquid, great for those of you who cannot take pills.

2. **Product made by:** Wyeth
   Product name: Centrum Silver
   We recommend: One pill, once a day
   Where to purchase: Just about any pharmacy, grocery store or vitamin store nationwide

   Note: This product is actually better for adults of all ages than the standard Centrum product, so don't worry if you're less than fifty years old. There are no megadoses of any vitamins or minerals in this product. If you're worried about the possible side effects of oversupplementation, this is the product for you.

3. **Product made by:** The Vitamin Shoppe
   Product name: Liquid Multi
   We recommend: One capful (1 ounce), once a day
   Where to purchase: *www.thevitaminshoppe.com,* or any Vitamin Shoppe store

4. **Product made by:** GNC
   Product name: Ultra Mega Green
   We recommend: Three pills per day; you may take all three pills at once even though the labeling says to take one pill with each meal.
   Where to purchase: *www.GNC.com,* or any GNC store

5. **Product made by:** The Vitamin Shoppe
   Product name: One Daily
   We recommend: One pill, once a day
   Where to purchase: *www.thevitaminshoppe.com,* or any Vitamin Shoppe store

Calcium with magnesium and vitamin D

1. **Product made by:** Carlson Laboratories
   Product name: Liquid Cal-Mag
   We recommend: Two tablets, twice a day, for a total of four tablets per day
   Where to purchase: Available at most major vitamin stores or call Carlson direct at 1-888-234-5656, or log on to *www.carlsonlabs.com*

   Note: This product also contains vitamin D even though this fact is not clear from the name.

2. **Product made by:** Solaray
   Product name: Cal-Mag Citrate with Vitamin D
   We recommend: Three tablets, twice a day, for a total of six tablets per day
   Where to purchase: *www.thevitaminshoppe.com,* or any Vitamin Shoppe store

3. **Product made by:** Schiff
   Product name: Super Calcium-Magnesium with Vitamin D and Boron
   We recommend: Take one tablet at breakfast time with your multivitamin, then take two tablets at lunch for a total of three tablets per day
   Where to purchase: *www.thevitaminshoppe.com,* or any Vitamin Shoppe store, or major vitamin shop or drugstore nationwide

Natural vitamin E with selenium

1. **Product made by:** Solaray
   Product name: Bio E with Selenium
   We recommend: Two tablets per day, take both at once
   Where to purchase: *www.thevitaminshoppe.com,* or any Vitamin Shoppe store

Note: This product contains 100 percent natural vitamin E.

2. **Product made by:** Twin Lab

   Product name: Super E Caps Plus Selenium

   We recommend: One tablet per day

   Where to purchase: *www.twinlab.com,* or almost any major vitamin store nationwide, including the Vitamin Shoppe

   Note: This product also contains 100 percent natural vitamin E.

3. **Product made by:** The Vitamin Shoppe

   Product name: E-400 IU Plus Selenium 200 mcg

   We recommend: Take one tablet per day

   Where to purchase: *www.thevitaminshoppe.com* or any Vitamin Shoppe store

   Note: Again, this product contains 100 percent natural vitamin E.

Vitamin C with bioflavonoids

1. **Product made by:** Solgar

   Product name: HY-C

   We recommend: Two tablets per day, one with breakfast and one with lunch

   Where to purchase: *www.solgar.com,* or locate a retailer near you by calling 1-877-SOLGAR-4

2. **Product made by:** The Vitamin Shoppe

   Product name: C-500 Complex

   We recommend: Two tablets per day, one with breakfast and one with lunch

   Where to purchase: *www.thevitaminshoppe.com,* or any Vitamin Shoppe store

GLA (from evening primrose oil)

1. **Product made by:** Barlean's Organic Oils

   Product name: Barlean's Organic Evening Primrose Oil

   We recommend: Although the labeling suggests taking two soft gels per day, you only need to take one soft gel per day to get 130 mg of GLA. However, individuals with inflammation-mediated conditions may want to take two or even three soft gels daily.

   Where to purchase: *www.barleans.com,* or try your local natural foods store

   Note: This is a superior-quality product from a superior company.

Fish oil (containing EPA and DHA)

1. **Product made by:** Nordic Naturals

   Product name: Ultimate Omega

   We recommend: Take two soft gels every day

   Where to purchase: Many health food and vitamin stores, or try *www.nordicnaturals.com,* or call 1-800-662-2544

   Note: This is another very high quality product. Most fish oil products contain too little EPA and too little DHA. Just two Ultimate Omega soft gels contain all the omega-3 fish oil you need for optimum health.

Supplements for Children

Children twelve years old and under will benefit from taking a daily multivitamin and a daily essential fat supplement. Children do not need to take all of the higher-dose supplements we recommend to adults.

Daily Vitamin Planner for Children

Take at Breakfast

Multivitamin, multimineral supplement

Take at Dinner

ProEFA Liquid essential fat supplement

Supplement Shopping Guide for Children

There is no need to limit your selection to these particular products. These recommendations are provided only as suggestions. Many children prefer the taste and consistency of alternative products. What's most important is that your children take their vitamins. Again, we highly recommend your children also take an essential fat supplement for optimal health and growth.

Multivitamin, multimineral supplement

1. **Product made by:** Northwest Natural Products

   Product name: L'il Critters Gummy Vites

   We recommend: Children ages 2 through 12 should take two gummy bear vitamins per day.

   Where to purchase: *www.gummybearvitamins.com,* or purchase at popular drugstores, discount stores and grocery stores nationwide

2. **Product made by:** Wyeth

   Product name: "Centrum Kids Rugrats Extra Calcium"

   We recommend: Children between 2 and 4 years old should take one-half tablet daily. Children ages 4 through 12 years old should take one tablet daily.

Where to purchase: Most major drugstores, grocery stores or vitamin stores nationwide

Note: This product is obviously a better choice if your children avoid dairy products. Calcium takes up quite a bit of space so it's difficult to put large amounts of calcium into a convenient children's supplement.

Essential fat supplement (containing GLA, EPA and DHA)

1. **Product made by:** Nordic Naturals

   Product name: ProEFA Liquid

   We recommend: Children under the age of 4 should take ¼ teaspoon daily. Children ages 4 through 12 should take ½ teaspoon daily.

   Where to purchase: Many health food and vitamin stores, or try *www.nordicnaturals.com*, or call 1-800-662-2544

   Note: Remember, children need essential fats every bit as much, if not more, than you do. Children have a difficult time swallowing pills so we recommend this liquid supplementation for them. Nordic Naturals liquid oils are very pure and very fresh. There's not even a hint of fishy aftertaste. This product contains a small amount of vitamin E to preserve its freshness.

Part Four

The Gold Coast Cookbook

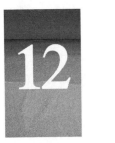

12 Breakfast and Brunch

Chunky Apple-Raisin Morning Muffins

YIELDS 12 MUFFINS

1.5 GRAMS SATURATED FAT PER SERVING

Ingredients

Canola oil cooking spray

¾ cup whole wheat flour

⅓ cup ground flaxseeds
  (we recommend Barlean's Forti-Flax)

2 tablespoons wheat germ

1 teaspoon baking powder

1 teaspoon baking soda

2 teaspoons cinnamon

½ teaspoon nutmeg

2 tablespoons brown sugar

¼ cup Splenda all-natural sugar
  substitute

1 cup unsweetened applesauce

2 tablespoons high-oleic canola oil

2 tablespoons butter, melted

1 egg

2 Granny Smith apples, chopped
  (no need to peel)

½ cup golden raisins

½ cup walnuts, chopped

Method

1. Preheat oven to 400 degrees and spray muffin tins with canola oil cooking spray.

2. In a medium bowl, mix the flour, flaxseeds, wheat germ, baking powder, baking soda, cinnamon, nutmeg, brown sugar and Splenda.

3. In a separate bowl, blend the applesauce, canola oil, butter and egg; then mix the wet ingredients in with the dry.

4. Add apples, raisins and walnuts to the batter and blend well. Transfer the batter to muffin tins and bake for 25 minutes. Muffins are done when a toothpick inserted in the middle comes out clean.

5. Let muffins cool completely before serving.

Chef's Notes

Reminiscent of a spice cake, these muffins satisfy a sweet tooth without sacrificing nutrition (they even contain omega-3-rich flaxseeds). Serve for breakfast with a tablespoon of all-natural peanut butter or almond butter and a cup of milk, soy milk or yogurt.

Dutch-Apple Pancakes

SERVES 2

2.5 GRAMS SATURATED FAT PER SERVING

Ingredients

1 whole apple, cored and sliced into rings
Cinnamon, to taste
1 teaspoon butter
⅓ cup Hodgson Mill brand Insta-Bake Whole Wheat Variety Baking Mix
3 tablespoons ground flaxseeds (we recommend Barlean's Forti-Flax)
1 packet Splenda sugar substitute

1 egg plus 1 egg white (keep the egg whites separate from the egg yolk)
⅓ cup 2% milk plus 2 tablespoons
¼ teaspoon pure vanilla extract
Canola oil cooking spray
Powdered sugar

Method

1. Sprinkle both sides of the apple slices with cinnamon.

2. Melt 1 teaspoon butter in a large nonstick skillet over medium heat. Sauté apple slices 2 to 3 minutes on each side or until apples are tender but not too soft. Transfer the apples to a separate plate and set aside.

3. Mix the Insta-Bake Whole Wheat Variety Baking Mix, ground flaxseeds, Splenda and milk in a large bowl; beat in the egg yolk, cinnamon and the vanilla extract.

4. Beat the two egg whites until stiff. Slowly add to the batter a little at a time, stirring well after each addition.

5. Spray skillet with canola oil cooking spray and arrange a few apple slices in the skillet about 2 inches apart. Ladle some of the batter over each apple slice to make a pancake. Cook each pancake about 2 to 3 minutes (or until small bubbles start to form), turn and cook another 2 to 3 minutes until pancake is done. Serve immediately.

Chef's Notes

Pancakes are always a family favorite on Sunday mornings. Serve with a tiny bit of powdered sugar and a glass of low-fat milk.

No-Fuss Baked Banana French Toast Casserole

Ingredients

Canola oil cooking spray

4 pieces whole-grain bread
(such as Alvarado Street Bakery California
Style Complete Protein Bread)

2 bananas, thinly sliced into rounds

Cinnamon, to taste

¼ cup plus 1 tablespoon ground flaxseeds
(we recommend Barlean's Forti-Flax)

¾ cup soy milk or low-fat milk

2 eggs plus 1 egg white

1 teaspoon pure vanilla extract

2 packets Splenda sugar substitute

¼ cup nut butter of choice

Method

1. Preheat the oven to 425 degrees. Spray the bottom and sides of an 8-x-8-inch square baking dish with canola oil cooking spray.

2. Tear bread into bite-size pieces and loosely arrange in two layers on the bottom of the baking dish. Lay the banana slices on top of the bread, season with a generous amount of cinnamon. Sprinkle the flaxseeds evenly on top.

3. In a medium-sized bowl, mix the soy milk, eggs, egg white, vanilla extract and Splenda and beat well. Pour the mixture evenly over the bananas and bread.

4. Bake for 20 minutes. Allow French toast to cool and set for 10 minutes before serving. Spread nut butter evenly over the top and serve.

Chef's Notes

This recipe came about after the fifth day in a row our toddler asked for French toast. I just threw all of the same ingredients I used to make his French toast (I usually coat the bread with flaxseed after dipping it in the eggs) into a casserole dish and baked it. It is super quick and easy to make, and it tastes wonderful. You can make it ahead, refrigerate it and serve it for up to 4 days (to re-serve, heat it in the microwave for about 1 minute).

Nutty Carrot Raisin Bread *(or Muffins)*

SERVES 9 (MAKES 9 MUFFINS)

0 GRAMS SATURATED FAT PER SERVING

Ingredients

Canola oil cooking spray

2 eggs, beaten

¼ cup high-oleic canola oil

¼ cup honey

¼ cup unsweetened applesauce

1 teaspoon pure vanilla extract

1 cup whole wheat flour

2 tablespoons wheat germ

¼ cup ground flaxseeds
    (we recommend Barlean's Forti-Flax)

¼ cup Splenda sugar substitute

½ teaspoon ground cloves

½ teaspoon cinnamon

½ teaspoon baking powder

½ teaspoon baking soda

1 cup shredded carrots

½ cup raisins

½ cup chopped pecans

Method

1. Preheat the oven to 350 degrees. Spray an 8½-x-4½-inch loaf pan or a 12-cup muffin tin with canola oil cooking spray.

2. In a small bowl, beat the eggs. Mix in the oil, honey, applesauce and vanilla extract.

3. In a large bowl, combine the flour, wheat germ, ground flaxseeds, Splenda, ground cloves, cinnamon, baking powder and baking soda. Add the liquid ingredients to the dry ingredients and stir until well blended. Mix in the carrots, raisins and pecans.

4. To make bread: Pour batter into prepared pan and bake for 45 minutes.

   To make muffins: Pour batter into prepared muffin tin and bake for 20 to 25 minutes.

5. When done, remove from pan or muffin tin and cool on a wire rack.

Chef's Notes

Serve these muffins for breakfast, snack or even at a luncheon. They are simple to make, delicious to eat and healthy.

Raspberries & Cream Soy Smoothie

SERVES 2

0 GRAMS SATURATED FAT PER SERVING

Ingredients

1 cup soy milk or low-fat milk

8 ounces silken tofu

(or ½ package of Nasoya Silken Tofu)

1½ cups frozen raspberries, semithawed

3 tablespoons ground flaxseeds

(we recommend Barlean's Forti-Flax)

2–3 packets Splenda sugar substitute

1 teaspoon pure almond extract

Method

Toss all of the ingredients into a blender and whip until smooth and creamy, about 1 minute.

Chef's Notes

Smoothies are a wonderful way to introduce tofu to your diet. This recipe is so delicious you won't believe you're eating tofu (neither will your kids, so don't tell them!).

Spinach, Cheese & Tofu Quiche with Easy Crust

SERVES 6

5.5 GRAMS SATURATED FAT PER SERVING

Ingredients

Crust:

1 cup whole-wheat flour
¾ cup ground flaxseeds
  (we recommend Barlean's Forti-Flax)
½ cup wheat germ
½ teaspoon salt
3 tablespoons butter, cold
2 teaspoons lemon juice
3 tablespoons ice water

Filling:

7 ounces extra-firm tofu, drained
  and patted dry with paper towels
¾ cup low-fat shredded mozzarella cheese
Salt, to taste
White pepper, to taste
½ teaspoon nutmeg, divided
4 eggs, beaten
10 ounces frozen chopped spinach,
  thawed and thoroughly patted dry with
  paper towels

Method

Crust:

1. Preheat the oven to 450 degrees.

2. In a medium-sized bowl, combine the flour, ground flaxseeds, wheat germ and salt.

3. Cut the butter into the flour mixture with two knives. Use your fingers to mix in the butter until the mixture resembles coarse crumbs and the butter is well blended. Add the lemon juice and water and mix thoroughly. Chill for 5 minutes in the freezer.

4. Press the crumbs onto the bottom and up the sides of a 9-inch pie plate. Bake for 8 minutes. Remove the crust from the oven and set aside.

Filling:

1. Crumble the tofu, Lay the tofu and shredded cheese on the bottom of the prebaked pie crust. Season with salt, white pepper and half of the measured nutmeg.

2. In a medium-sized bowl, beat the eggs, then mix in the spinach. Season with salt and white pepper and the remaining measured nutmeg.

3. Pour the spinach and egg mixture over the cheese and tofu and bake for 15 minutes. Reduce the heat to 350 degrees and bake for an additional 10 minutes. Allow to cool for several minutes before slicing and serving.

Chef's Notes

Serve this quiche for brunch with a side of fresh fruit salad or fresh tomato salsa.

Vegetable & Salmon Frittata

SERVES 4

3.5 GRAMS SATURATED FAT PER SERVING

Ingredients

1 tablespoon extra-virgin olive oil

1 Spanish onion, chopped

1 red bell pepper, chopped

Salt, to taste

4 large eggs

1 tablespoon low-fat milk

2 tablespoons low-fat sour cream

Fresh salsa, for garnish

¼ teaspoon coarsely ground black pepper

¼ cup low-fat feta cheese, crumbled

1 cup frozen corn kernels, thawed

¾ cup canned salmon, drained

3 tablespoons chopped scallions, both white and green parts

2 tablespoons freshly grated Parmesan cheese

Method

1. Preheat oven to 400 degrees. Lightly grease an 8-inch springform pan or a 10-inch pie plate.

2. Heat a small pan over medium-high heat and add the oil. When the oil is hot, add the onion. Sauté for 5 minutes or until onion is translucent. Add the bell pepper and cook until soft, about 5 more minutes. Season with salt to taste and spread the vegetables out on the bottom of the prepared pan.

3. In a medium-sized bowl, whisk together the eggs, milk, sour cream and pepper. Mix in the feta cheese, corn kernels, salmon and scallions. Season the egg mixture with a bit of salt. Pour the mixture on top of the vegetables.

4. Bake for 18 to 20 minutes. Sprinkle with the Parmesan cheese and cook for 3 more minutes, or until the cheese is melted, forming a glaze. Allow the frittata to cool, then slice and serve warm with fresh salsa.

Chef's Notes

Filling and delicious, this recipe is great for breakfast, brunch or even dinner. Use omega-3 eggs (such as Egglands Best) and this already healthy dish will be just that much healthier.

13 Dressings, Dips, Soups and Salads

Amazing Apple Vinaigrette

SERVES 12

0 GRAMS SATURATED FAT PER SERVING

Ingredients

1 handful of fresh parsley

¼ cup flaxseed oil (we recommend Barlean's brand)

½ cup unsweetened applesauce

¼ cup apple juice

1 tablespoon brown sugar

¼ cup apple cider vinegar

2 garlic cloves, chopped

¼ teaspoon salt

Method

Toss all ingredients into a blender or food processor and puree until smooth and creamy. Serve with mixed greens.

Note: *You can store this vinaigrette in a covered container in the refrigerator for up to 2 days.*

Chef's Notes

Your friends will be clamoring for the secret ingredient because this recipe really lives up to its name: Amazing!

Honey Lovin' Lime Vinaigrette

SERVES 4

0 GRAMS SATURATED FAT PER SERVING

Ingredients

¼ cup flaxseed oil (we recommend
Barlean's brand)
3 tablespoons fresh lime juice
1 tablespoon honey

1 teaspoon crushed garlic cloves
⅛ teaspoon grated lime peel
⅛ teaspoon salt

Method

Combine all of the ingredients in a medium-size cup and whisk with a fork. The flavor of the dressing will intensify if you allow the vinaigrette to sit in a covered container in the refrigerator for about half an hour before serving.

Note: *You can store this vinaigrette in a covered container in the refrigerator for up to 2 days.*

Chef's Notes

An unusual and delicate dressing, this vinaigrette is sensational on a salad of mixed greens, freshly sliced tomatoes, grilled chicken strips, a bit of freshly shaved Parmesan cheese and "croutons" made of crushed tortilla chips (we use all-natural Kettle Blue Corn variety). Go easy on the tortilla chips and use no more than a small handful on each salad.

Cilantro & Key Lime Vinaigrette

SERVES 4

0 GRAMS SATURATED FAT PER SERVING

Ingredients

1½ cups fresh cilantro (loosely packed)

2 garlic cloves, chopped

¼ cup fresh lime juice

1 tablespoon all-natural peanut butter

¼ cup flaxseed oil (we recommend Barlean's brand)

2 tablespoons honey

⅛ teaspoon salt

Method

Toss all ingredients into a blender or food processor and blend for about 1 minute or until dressing is smooth and creamy.

Note: *You can store this vinaigrette in a covered container in the refrigerator for up to 2 days.*

Chef's Notes

Think beyond salad greens and try this versatile dressing mixed with white beans, on top of grilled fish, or tossed with whole grain pasta, grilled chicken or shrimp, and roasted vegetables (such as red peppers).

Sesame Garlic Dressing

SERVES 4

0 GRAMS SATURATED FAT PER SERVING

Ingredients

3 tablespoons flaxseed oil (we recommend Barlean's brand)

2 tablespoons tahini (sesame seed butter)

¼ cup chopped parsley

2 garlic cloves

1 tablespoon soy sauce

2 tablespoons fresh lemon juice

1 tablespoon balsamic vinegar

2 tablespoons apple juice

1 teaspoon honey

Method

Toss all ingredients into a blender or food processor and blend well for about 1 minute or until dressing is smooth and creamy.

Note: *You can store this vinaigrette in a covered container in the refrigerator for up to 2 days.*

Chef's Notes

Serve this dressing over fresh mixed salad greens garnished with chopped hard-boiled egg, cooked corn kernels and toasted sesame seeds.

Lemon Cashew Dip

SERVES 4

1 GRAM SATURATED FAT PER SERVING

Ingredients

1 cup cashews
¼ cup fresh lemon juice
1 tablespoon canola-oil mayonnaise
2 tablespoons light sour cream
1 teaspoon brown sugar
2 tablespoons water

Method

Toss all of the ingredients into a food processor or blender; process for 1 to 2 minutes on high, or until creamy and smooth.

Note: *You can store this dip in a covered container in the refrigerator for up to 2 days.*

Chef's Notes

This tasty dip is perfect with skewer-grilled chicken or pork. It is also a wonderful veggie dip. Try dipping red bell peppers, celery, carrots, endive leafs, broccoli, cauliflower and so on.

Ricotta and Honey Fruit Dip with Mint

SERVES 10

2.5 GRAMS SATURATED FAT PER SERVING

Ingredients

½ cup whipped cream cheese

½ cup low-fat ricotta cheese

3 tablespoons honey

1 tablespoon Splenda sugar substitute

¼ cup light sour cream

2 tablespoons fresh lemon juice

¼ cup packed fresh mint leaves

Method

In a food processor or blender, blend all ingredients until smooth and creamy, about 1 minute. Transfer to a covered container and refrigerate until serving time.

Note: *You can store this dip in a covered container in the refrigerator for up to 2 days.*

Chef's Notes

Serve this easy-to-make dip with fresh fruit on skewers. Try kiwi, grapes, melon, strawberries and pineapple.

South American Avocado Dip

SERVES 8

0 GRAMS SATURATED FAT PER SERVING

Ingredients

2 dark ripe avocados (save the seeds)

3 to 4 tablespoons *fresh* lime juice

2 tablespoons canola-oil mayonnaise

4 hard-boiled eggs, whites only

½ teaspoon Tabasco or other hot sauce

½ teaspoon salt

2 tablespoons chopped pimentos,
  drained and patted dry

Method

1. In a medium-sized bowl, mash the avocados; mix in the lime juice and canola-oil mayonnaise.

2. Chop the hard-boiled egg whites and combine with the avocado mixture. Season with Tabasco, salt and pimentos. Add the avocado seeds to the dip to prevent the avocado from turning color.

3. Cover with plastic wrap and keep refrigerated. Serve cold.

Chef's Notes

This is our version of the avocado dip given to us by a family friend. If you like avocados and limes, you'll be in heaven. Avocado dip is especially great on whole-grain crackers.

Zesty Peanut Butter Dip

SERVES 8 TO 12

1 GRAM SATURATED FAT PER SERVING

Ingredients

¾ cup all-natural peanut butter

1 cup silken tofu (before measuring, drain on paper towels and blot dry with a paper towel)

½ cup scallion stalks, coarsely chopped

1 cup chopped *fresh* cilantro

2 tablespoons brown sugar

3 tablespoons soy sauce

Juice from 2 limes

2 tablespoons apple cider vinegar

3 cloves garlic, chopped

Method

Combine all of the ingredients in a food processor and blend until almost smooth (flecks of green should still remain).

Chef's Notes

This dip is an excellent accompaniment to crudités. When serving crudités there are two things to keep in mind: (1) serve only the absolute freshest vegetables available, and (2) pay careful attention to the presentation of the vegetables and spend an extra minute or two on artful display. Cut your veggies into unique shapes and/or use special knives to make pretty patterns. We like carrots, cucumbers, cauliflower, endives, asparagus, celery and red peppers with this dip. For a heartier appetizer, try dipping kebabs of grilled chicken, pork, shrimp and even tofu.

Creamy Carrot & Red Pepper Soup

SERVES 10

1.5 GRAMS SATURATED FAT PER SERVING

Ingredients

1 tablespoon butter

1 tablespoon extra-virgin olive oil

2 cups onion, diced

1 red bell pepper, chopped

1 pound carrots, thinly sliced

2 teaspoons *dried* dill

Dash of salt, to taste

1 teaspoon white pepper

1 handful *fresh* dill, chopped

Juice from ½ lemon

3 cups all-natural chicken broth

8 ounces silken tofu (drained on a paper towel and patted dry)

1 cup whole milk

2 tablespoons light sour cream

Method

1. Mix the butter and extra-virgin olive oil in a large soup pot. When the butter has melted, add the onion, red pepper, carrots, dried dill and a dash of salt. Cover and cook over medium heat, stirring occasionally until the onion has softened completely (about 10 minutes).

2. Add 1 teaspoon white pepper, fresh dill, lemon juice and chicken broth. Bring to a boil, then simmer (partially covered) for 10 minutes. When done, remove the soup pot from the heat and let cool.

3. When soup is somewhat cool, toss all of the ingredients into a food processor or blender and blend until smooth.

4. Transfer liquid back to the soup pot, then add the tofu, milk and sour cream into the blender and blend until smooth.

5. Slowly add the tofu, milk and sour cream to the soup pot and simmer for another 5 to 10 minutes. Serve warm.

Chef's Notes

Creamy vegetable soups are a wonderful way to sneak tofu into your diet. Tofu has such a bland flavor that it's simply undetectable in a cream-based soup, promise!

Gold Coast Clam Chowder

SERVES 10

0.5 GRAMS SATURATED FAT PER SERVING

Ingredients

1 tablespoon extra-virgin olive oil

1 onion, finely chopped

5 garlic gloves, finely chopped

Six 6½-ounce cans chopped clams (drain well)

Salt, to taste

White pepper, to taste

Tabasco or other hot sauce, to taste

1 box (32 ounces) Pacific brand Creamy Organic Tomato Soup

1 jar (26 ounces) high-quality marinara sauce (we like San Marzano or Rao's brand)

1 cup whole milk

Method

1. In a large soup pot heat the extra-virgin olive oil over medium-high heat; add the onions and garlic and sauté several minutes until onions are soft.

2. Add *drained* clams, salt, white pepper and Tabasco to taste; sauté several minutes.

3. Add the tomato soup, marinara sauce and milk; simmer for 10 to 12 minutes.

4. Serve warm.

Chef's Notes

This is one of the easiest and best-tasting clam chowders you will find; friends and family are always asking for the recipe. It's a cross between Manhattan clam chowder and New England clam chowder. By making use of high-quality premade soup and tomato sauce you drastically reduce the preparation time without sacrificing flavor. Make a complete meal by adding a side salad, whole-grain rolls and fresh corn on the cob.

Spicy Curried Pumpkin Soup

SERVES 10

1.75 GRAMS SATURATED FAT PER SERVING

Ingredients

1 tablespoon butter

1 tablespoon extra-virgin olive oil

1 large onion, sliced

1 large Granny Smith apple, peeled and sliced

2½ cups all-natural chicken broth

2½ cups apple cider

1 cup *silken* tofu (drained well and patted as dry as possible with paper towels)

32 ounces canned pumpkin

½ cup whole milk

2 tablespoons heavy cream

½ teaspoon white pepper

Salt, to taste

2 teaspoons curry powder (or more to taste)

1 tablespoon brown sugar

Method

1. Heat the extra-virgin olive oil and butter in a large soup pot until butter melts, add the onion and apple and sauté until soft (do not brown).

2. Transfer the onion-apple mixture to a food processor or blender, add a small amount of the chicken broth and blend until smooth. Gradually add the remaining chicken broth and process until creamy, then pour *half* of the mixture into the soup pot.

3. Add the apple cider to the food processor and blend well. Then pour *half* of the mixture into the soup pot.

4. To the blender or food processor add the silken tofu and puree until smooth.

5. Transfer all of the contents from the food processor or blender to the soup pot. Heat the soup pot over medium heat and add canned pumpkin, milk, heavy cream, white pepper, salt, curry and brown sugar to the saucepan. Bring soup to a simmer for 5 minutes. Serve warm.

Chef's Notes

A perfect soup for fall, it is warm, flavorful and antioxidant-rich.

Caesar's Salad

SERVES 4

1.5 GRAMS SATURATED FAT PER SERVING

Ingredients

2 anchovy filets (optional)

1 tablespoon garlic cloves, crushed

½ cup canola-oil mayonnaise (purchase at natural foods store)

2 tablespoons grated Romano or Parmesan cheese (plus extra for garnish)

3 tablespoons fresh lemon juice

1 tablespoon flaxseed oil (we recommend Barlean's brand)

1 tablespoon Dijon mustard

1 teaspoon Worcestershire sauce

1 bag romaine lettuce (torn into bite-sized pieces)

Whole-wheat croutons (see Chef's Notes below)

Cherry tomatoes for garnish

½ cup grated Romano or Parmesan cheese

Freshly ground black pepper

Method

1. In a large bowl, mash anchovies with a fork. Add crushed garlic and blend until smooth.

2. Whisk in mayonnaise, then add the cheese, lemon juice, flaxseed oil, mustard and Worcestershire sauce. Whisk until smooth.

3. Tear the lettuce leaves into bite-size pieces and toss in dressing to lightly coat lettuce leaves. (Don't drown the lettuce leaves in the dressing, please!)

4. Garnish with whole-wheat croutons, cherry tomatoes, a little extra shredded Romano or Parmesan cheese and ground black pepper.

Chef's Notes

Make your own healthy and tasty whole-grain croutons by breaking whole-grain bread into bite-sized squares (minus the crust) and sautéing the crustless squares in extra-virgin olive oil, a bit of salt, a dash of Parmesan cheese and minced garlic until crispy.

Mixed Salad Greens with Pear and Feta Cheese

SERVES 4

3 GRAMS SATURATED FAT PER SERVING

Ingredients

Vinaigrette
2 tablespoons apple cider vinegar
½ cup flaxseed oil (we recommend Barlean's brand)
1 tablespoon honey
2 teaspoons Dijon mustard
½ teaspoon salt
½ teaspoon black pepper

Salad
8 cups mixed salad greens (buy prewashed and precut to save time)
2 ripe pears, sliced into lengthwise strips
½ cup coarsely chopped pecans, divided
4 ounces light feta cheese, crumbled

Method

1. In a small bowl, whisk the vinegar, flaxseed oil, honey, mustard, salt and pepper.

2. In a large bowl toss the salad greens, pear slices, pecans and feta cheese. Add vinaigrette to taste.

3. Serve immediately.

Note: *Store unused vinaigrette in a covered container in the refrigerator for up to 2 days.*

Chef's Notes

This is a great dish to serve to guests; it is simple to prepare, has a beautiful presentation and tastes fabulous. You may also want to serve it as a main course with whole-grain bread and grilled chicken strips.

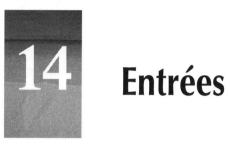

14 Entrées

Curried Apple-Turkey Burgers

SERVES 7

2 GRAMS SATURATED FAT PER SERVING

Ingredients

1¼ pounds extra-lean ground turkey

2 Granny Smith apples, diced (leave skin on; use an apple corer for speedy prep)

2 teaspoons curry powder

½ teaspoon salt

½ teaspoon pepper

1 tablespoon sesame seed butter (also known as tahini)

1 egg

1 tablespoon honey

¼ cup wheat germ

2 avocados

Method

1. Preheat the broiler.

2. Mix all of the ingredients, except the avocados, in a big bowl.

3. Use your hands to form the mixture into about seven medium-sized burgers. Place the burgers on a broiler pan about 2½ to 3 inches from the broiler. Broil for 3 to 5 minutes per side, or until thoroughly cooked.

4. Top burgers with avocado slices.

Chef's Notes

If in the past you've shunned conventional turkey burgers as tasteless, you're in for a pleasant surprise.

Far Eastern Tofu & Vegetable Stir Fry

SERVES 4

2 GRAMS SATURATED FAT PER SERVING

Ingredients

1 package extra-firm tofu (14 ounces)
1 tablespoon soy sauce
1 tablespoon lime juice
1 tablespoon white wine
1 tablespoon honey
1 tablespoon butter
1 tablespoon extra-virgin olive oil

1 medium red onion, quartered and sliced thin
3 cups shredded carrots
1 pound snow peas, stringed
2 tablespoons minced scallions, white parts only
1 tablespoon garlic, minced
1 tablespoon fresh gingerroot, minced

Special Sauce: Mix the following ingredients
• 2 tablespoons cider vinegar
• 1 tablespoon lime juice
• 1 tablespoon soy sauce
• 1 tablespoon brown sugar

Method

1. Drain tofu, pat dry with paper towels, and cut into ¾-inch cubes. Sandwich tofu between paper towels and set a weighted flat pan on top, allowing it to drain for at least 10 minutes.

2. While tofu is draining, mix soy sauce, lime juice, wine and honey in a medium bowl; toss tofu in the mixture and set aside (tossing occasionally).

3. Heat a medium-size, nonstick skillet over high heat for 2 to 3 minutes, and then add butter. Allow butter to melt (tip the pan so butter spreads evenly over the bottom). Drain the tofu from the marinade and add it to the buttered hot pan and lightly brown on all sides (about 5 minutes); scrape cooked tofu into a bowl and cover to keep warm.

4. Let pan heat back up for 1 minute, then drizzle 1 teaspoon extra-virgin olive oil onto the pan and add onion. Stir-fry onion for 2 minutes. Add the shredded carrots and stir fry for another minute. Drizzle another teaspoon of extra-virgin olive oil onto the onions and carrots and then add snow peas; stir fry for an additional minute.

5. Clear the center of the pan and add minced scallions, garlic and ginger; drizzle with 1 teaspoon extra-virgin olive oil and mash the scallions, garlic, and ginger onto the pan with the back of a spatula. Allow to cook for 30 seconds. Remove the pan from the heat and stir scallions, garlic and ginger mixture in with the vegetables.

6. Return pan to the heat and add the cooked tofu; stir in the "special sauce" until all ingredients are well coated and sauce is sizzling hot. Serve immediately.

Chef's Notes

Serve with a side of brown rice.

Filet Mignon with Garlic and Herb Puree

SERVES 4

4 GRAMS SATURATED FAT PER SERVING

Ingredients

2 very large garlic bulbs

3 teaspoons extra-virgin olive oil, divided

Salt, to taste

Ground pepper, to taste

1 tablespoon light cream

1 teaspoon balsamic vinegar

2 tablespoons water

3 tablespoons chopped fresh parsley

4 (5-ounce) filet mignons, 1½ to 2 inches thick, meticulously trimmed of all visible fat

Method

To make garlic and herb puree:

1. Preheat the oven to 300 degrees. Remove the loose, papery outer skins of the garlic, leaving the garlic bulbs intact. Use a small knife to slice off the top ¼ inch of each clove. Place each garlic bulb, cut side up, on a 12-inch square of aluminum foil.

2. Drizzle 1 teaspoon of the oil on top of each bulb and season to taste with salt and pepper. Fold the aluminum foil to make a closed "package" and set the packages in a small baking dish. Roast the bulbs for 30 minutes. Remove the bulbs from the foil and roast for an additional 45 minutes.

3. Let the garlic bulbs cool and then slip the cloves out of their skins and transfer to a food processor or blender. Add one teaspoon of oil, light cream, balsamic vinegar, water and parsley. Puree until smooth and season with salt and pepper to taste.

To make filet mignon:

1. Season the beef on both sides with salt and pepper and then spread half of the prepared garlic and herb butter on the tops of each piece of meat.

2. Place filets on broiler pan as close to heat as possible and broil to desired doneness (about 2 to 4 minutes per side).

3. Serve immediately with the remaining garlic and herb puree spooned onto the tops of each portion.

Chef's Notes

The garlic enriches the flavor of the beef and provides culinary interest.

Garlicky Tomato Shrimp

SERVES 4

1.5 GRAMS SATURATED FAT PER SERVING

Ingredients

1 tablespoon extra-virgin olive oil

2 teaspoons butter

2 cups finely chopped Spanish onions

2 whole red peppers, finely chopped

¼ cup garlic, finely chopped

1 teaspoon paprika

2 teaspoons cumin

1 (28-ounce) can whole,
   peeled tomatoes, drained

Tabasco, to taste

Salt, to taste

Black pepper, to taste

1½ pounds jumbo shrimp, peeled and
   de-veined

1 cup fresh cilantro, chopped

Method

1. Heat the oil and butter in a large nonstick skillet over medium heat. Add the onion, red and green pepper, garlic, paprika and cumin. Sauté for 2 to 3 minutes, mix in the tomatoes and mash them down with a potato masher. Season to taste with salt, pepper and a splash or two of Tabasco. Simmer for about 10 minutes or until mixture thickens and most of the liquid evaporates.

2. Add the shrimp and cook, turning occasionally, until the shrimp curls and is cooked through, about 5 to 6 minutes. Stir in the cilantro. Cook for just a few seconds, until cilantro begins to wilt. Remove the skillet from the heat.

3. Serve immediately.

Chef's Notes

Serve over a small mound of brown rice with a side of petite peas.

Grilled Lemon Sole with Pineapple Peach Salsa

SERVES 4

0 GRAMS SATURATED FAT PER SERVING

Ingredients

Salsa:

1 cup frozen peaches (thawed), finely chopped

1 cup fresh pineapple, finely chopped
(buy precut pineapple to save time)

½ cup red onion, finely chopped

½ cup fresh cilantro, finely chopped

1 tablespoon fresh lime juice

¼ cup orange juice

1 teaspoon flaxseed oil (we recommend
Barlean's brand)

1 teaspoon Tabasco or other hot sauce

1 teaspoon brown sugar

½ teaspoon chili powder

⅛ teaspoon salt

Fish:

1½ pounds lemon sole (or any mild
white fish such as flounder or tilapia)

Extra-virgin olive oil

Salt

Ground pepper

Method

Salsa:

Mix all of the ingredients for the salsa in a medium-sized bowl and then refrigerate for 20 minutes to allow flavors to meld.

Fish:

1. Heat a gas or charcoal grill to high.

2. Lightly oil the fish and season both sides with salt and pepper.

3. Use tongs to place the fish on the grill. Grill, turning once, until the fish is opaque in the center at its thickest part (about 5 minutes per side).

4. Place the fish on individual plates and spoon one-fourth of the salsa onto each piece of fish. Serve immediately.

Chef's Notes

If you don't want to use the grill, you can also sauté the fish in a nonstick skillet in a little bit of extra-virgin olive oil.

Grilled Tofu Kebabs with Rosemary-Lemon Yogurt Sauce

SERVES 4

1.75 GRAMS SATURATED FAT PER SERVING

Ingredients

Dipping sauce:

1 cup plain low-fat yogurt
3 tablespoons fresh minced rosemary
1 tablespoon minced garlic
1 tablespoon flaxseed oil
2 tablespoons fresh lemon juice

¼ cup light sour cream
½ teaspoon salt
¼ teaspoon white pepper
1 teaspoon sugar

Kebabs:

28 ounces extra-firm tofu, drained, patted dry and cut into 1-inch cubes
4 medium zucchini, cubed into bite-sized pieces
2 large onions, peeled and cut into bite-sized pieces
20 mushrooms, whole
1 tablespoon extra-virgin olive oil
Salt, to taste
White pepper, to taste
20 whole cherry tomatoes

Method

Dipping sauce:

Combine all of the ingredients for the dipping sauce in a medium-sized bowl and stir well. Cover and refrigerate until serving time.

Kebabs:

1. Blanch the onion in boiling water for 2 to 3 minutes and drain.

2. Alternate tofu, zucchini, onion and mushroom on skewers, always ending with mushrooms. Brush the vegetables and tofu with olive oil, and season with salt and pepper to taste.

3. Place tofu on the grill; cook for 8 to 10 minutes on each side.

4. Serve warm with cherry tomatoes and dipping sauce.

Chef's Notes

If you don't know what to do with tofu, kebabs are the perfect start. Kebabs are a breeze to make and visually appealing to eat. And of course they're tasty, too!

Lemon-Roasted Scallops with Artichokes

SERVES 4

0 GRAMS SATURATED FAT PER SERVING

Ingredients

Olive oil cooking spray

¼ cup whole-wheat bread crumbs

2 tablespoons wheat germ

3 teaspoons extra-virgin olive oil, divided

1½ pounds large sea scallops

1 (10-ounce) box of frozen artichoke hearts, thawed and chopped into 1-inch pieces

10 scallions, sliced into 1-inch segments

¼ cup dry white wine

Juice of ½ lemon (no seeds)

3 minced garlic cloves

¼ teaspoon salt

¼ teaspoon white pepper

½ teaspoon dried basil

Method

1. Preheat the oven to 400 degrees. Spray an 8-x-8-inch baking dish with nonstick cooking spray.

2. In a small bowl, mix the bread crumbs with the wheat germ and 1 teaspoon extra-virgin olive oil.

3. In a medium-size bowl, combine the scallops, artichoke hearts, remaining 2 teaspoons of olive oil, scallions, wine, lemon juice, garlic, salt, pepper and dried basil. Transfer scallop mixture to the baking dish and bake for 15 minutes.

4. Remove scallops from the oven and increase temperature to broil. Drain off any excess liquid from the baking dish and top the scallops with the wheat germ and bread crumbs.

5. Broil scallops for 8 minutes or until topping is deep gold.

Chef's Notes

Tasty lemon scallops are wonderful served with a simple side salad of mixed greens and roasted portobello mushrooms. Portobello mushrooms are rich tasting and easy to prepare. Simply slice mushrooms lengthwise and place in a baking pan; drizzle a bit of extra-virgin olive oil on top and toss in some scallions and salt. Then roast for about 8 minutes. The mushrooms can be roasted at the same time you are roasting the scallops. Finish off the meal with fresh berries and a small scoop of all-natural vanilla ice cream, or skip the ice cream and splash the fruit with apricot brandy.

Lime-Marinated Sea Bass with Chili-Spice Rub

SERVES 4

1 GRAM SATURATED FAT PER SERVING

Ingredients

4 (6-ounce) sea bass fillets (about 1 inch thick)
2 teaspoons extra-virgin olive oil

Marinade:

Juice from 4 whole limes
Juice from 4 whole lemons
4 teaspoons chili powder
7 cloves garlic, crushed
2 teaspoons hot sauce (such as Tabasco)

Spice rub:

2 teaspoons chili powder
4 teaspoons freshly ground black pepper
2 teaspoons ground cumin
4 teaspoons paprika
½ teaspoon salt

Method

1. To prepare the marinade, combine all of the marinade ingredients in a large ziplock plastic bag, then add the fish to the bag. Seal and marinate the fish in the refrigerator for about an hour. Remove fish from bag and discard marinade.

2. Meanwhile, prepare spice rub by combining all of the spice rub ingredients together in a small bowl. Mix with a spoon.

3. Rub the spice rub over the fish to coat both sides.

4. Heat the oil in a large nonstick skillet over medium-high heat. Add fish and cook approximately 6 minutes on each side or until the fish flakes easily on both sides when tested with a fork.

5. Serve immediately.

Chef's Notes

Moroccan inspired, this spicy fish recipe is wonderful with a side of black beans, roasted red peppers and roasted carrots.

Mint-Infused Leg of Lamb

SERVES 8

5 GRAMS SATURATED FAT PER SERVING

Ingredients

1 (4-pound) rolled boneless leg of lamb,
trimmed of all visible fat
(see instructions below)
Salt and freshly ground black pepper
1 cup fresh mint leaves

Juice from 2 whole lemons
¼ cup extra-virgin olive oil
½ cup mint jelly
3 garlic cloves, chopped
¼ cup unsweetened applesauce

Method

1. Unroll the roast and carefully trim all visible fat using both kitchen shears and a knife. Season both sides of the roast with salt and pepper.

2. In a food processor or blender, prepare the marinade by processing together the mint leaves, lemon juice, extra-virgin olive oil, mint jelly, garlic cloves and applesauce.

3. Pour three-fourths of the marinade over the roast (reserve the remaining marinade for later). Cover and marinate the roast for at least 6 hours (or overnight) in the refrigerator.

4. Remove the roast from the marinade. Reroll the roast and secure at 1-inch intervals with twine.

5. Preheat oven to 425 degrees.

6. Bake for 50 minutes or until a meat thermometer registers 145 degrees (medium-rare) or desired degree of doneness. Note: Lamb is usually best when pink inside and crusty outside. Let roast stand for 20 minutes before slicing.

7. Meanwhile, bring the reserved marinade to a boil for 2 minutes. Pour over the lamb just before serving.

Chef's Notes

Although lamb is perfect for Easter dinner, we enjoy it year-round. However, do take extra care to trim as much visible fat as possible from your roast.

Parsley & Nut-Crusted Baked Halibut

SERVES 4

1 GRAM SATURATED FAT PER SERVING

Ingredients

Olive oil or canola oil cooking spray
1½ pounds thin halibut fillets (or substitute
    another mild white fish such as cod,
    tilapia or catfish)
Salt, to taste
Black pepper, to taste

1½ cups very thinly sliced almonds
    (be sure they are thinly sliced
    and not slivered)
¼ cup fresh parsley
1 teaspoon butter, at room temperature
2 large eggs
4 lemon wedges

Method

1. Preheat the oven to 400 degrees. Thoroughly spray a baking dish with olive oil or canola oil cooking spray.

2. Cut fish into serving pieces, and blot dry with paper towels. Season both sides to taste with salt and pepper.

3. In a food processor, process the almonds with the parsley until finely chopped. Add the butter and pulse until combined.

4. Beat the eggs. Dredge both sides of the fish in the egg. Press the almond and parsley mixture on both sides of the fish firmly with your fingertips. Place fish in oiled baking pan and bake for 15 minutes or until cooked through and opaque at the thickest part (test with a knife).

5. Drizzle with lemon juice and serve immediately.

Chef's Notes

Nut-crusted fish recipes usually require frying in vegetable oil; our version is healthier, much less messy to prepare and (importantly) every bit as flavorful.

Parisian Vegetable Beef Stew

SERVES 6

4 GRAMS SATURATED FAT PER SERVING

Ingredients

1 teaspoon extra-virgin olive oil

1 large onion, chopped

1½ pounds lean beef stew meat (trimmed of all fat and cut into 1-inch cubes)

4 tablespoons whole-wheat flour

½ teaspoon salt

½ teaspoon white pepper

1 pound fresh button mushrooms (sliced)

1 cup dry vermouth wine

1½ cups fat-free, all-natural chicken broth

½ cup orange juice, divided

2 teaspoons dried basil

4 garlic cloves (crushed)

1 (15-ounce) can diced tomatoes, do not drain

1 package (or 1½ cups) frozen petite peas

1 package (or ½ cup) frozen corn

Method

1. Heat extra-virgin olive oil in a large wok over medium-high heat. Add onion and beef and sauté for 8 minutes, stirring occasionally.

2. Sprinkle the flour, salt and pepper over the beef mixture and cook for 1 minute more while stirring constantly.

3. Add the mushrooms, wine, chicken broth, half of the orange juice, basil, garlic cloves and tomatoes. Bring to a boil.

4. Reduce heat. Simmer, uncovered for 25 minutes (beef should be tender and mushrooms still slightly firm). Add the frozen peas and corn and the remaining half of the orange juice and simmer for an additional 5 minutes. Let cool slightly before serving; serve warm.

Chef's Notes

An effortless, one-dish meal; this stew is hearty and healthy with European flair. We actually had a great stew very similar to this on our honeymoon, and although the ingredients in this version obviously aren't exactly the same as the ones used at the Parisian café, the flavor does come pretty close.

Penne Pasta & Chicken Casserole
with Roasted Red Pepper Puree

SERVES 6

3 GRAMS SATURATED FAT PER SERVING

Ingredients

1½ pounds boneless, skinless chicken breasts, cut into bite-sized pieces

Salt (to taste)

White pepper (to taste)

Paprika (to taste)

1 tablespoon extra-virgin olive oil, plus 2 teaspoons for sautéing

6 cups tightly packed fresh spinach leaves, coarsely chopped

3 cups whole-wheat penne pasta, cooked al dente

Olive oil cooking spray

½ cup shredded Parmesan or Romano cheese

3 tablespoons Neufchatel cream cheese (or whipped cream cheese)

One 12-ounce jar roasted red peppers (packed in water), drained very well and patted dry with a cloth

Method

1. Preheat oven to 375 degrees and season all sides of the chicken with salt, white pepper and a generous amount of paprika.

2. Heat 2 teaspoons extra-virgin olive oil in a large soup pot over medium heat. Add seasoned chicken and pan sear on all sides until lightly browned (about 4 minutes).

3. Add the spinach leaves to the chicken and mix well. Cover the pot for a minute to allow the spinach to wilt. When spinach is almost wilted, add the pasta and toss well. Add a bit more white pepper and paprika.

4. Remove the chicken, spinach and pasta from the heat and spray a casserole dish with olive oil cooking spray; transfer the chicken, spinach and pasta to the casserole dish and sprinkle with Parmesan or Romano cheese.

5. Dot the top of the casserole dish with tiny dollops of cream cheese. Bake casserole for 20 minutes.

6. Meanwhile, prepare the roasted red pepper puree by blending the drained red peppers with 1 tablespoon extra-virgin olive oil. Season to taste with a bit of white pepper.

7. Remove casserole from oven, pour some of the sauce over casserole and place back in the oven for 5 to 10 more minutes. Remove casserole and serve at once.

Chef's Notes

An elegant one-dish meal, this is definitely not your typical casserole. The roasted red pepper puree is incredibly simple to prepare and adds a special gourmet touch.

Rising-Sun Gingered Salmon

SERVES 4

1 GRAM SATURATED FAT PER SERVING

Ingredients

¼ cup soy sauce

¼ cup plus 1 tablespoon lime juice

4 tablespoons brown sugar

¼ cup freshly grated ginger

3 tablespoons rice wine vinegar
  (or white vinegar)

1½ pounds of salmon steaks, cut
  into individual portions
  (about 1 inch thick)

5 scallions, thinly sliced

Method

1. In a large stainless-steel skillet mix the soy sauce, lime juice, brown sugar, grated ginger and vinegar.

2. Heat the sauce over medium-high heat. When the sauce is hot add the salmon, skin side down, and cover with a lid. Let the salmon cook for approximately 4 minutes, then carefully flip each portion and gently scrape off and discard the skin. Cover fish again and cook an additional 4 minutes. Flip the fish once more, cover and cook until done, about 3 more minutes.

3. When done, transfer fish to individual serving plates, drizzle generously with the ginger sauce, and garnish with sliced scallions.

Chef's Notes

True fusion cuisine, Gingered Salmon is an intriguing and exotic combination of Oriental flavors. Serve this salmon over a bed of whole-grain pasta and edamame beans.

Salmon Bake with
Creamy Lemon Mustard Sauce

SERVES 4

2 GRAMS SATURATED FAT PER SERVING

Ingredients

4 salmon filets, about 5 to 6 ounces each
Salt, to taste
White pepper, to taste
4 tablespoons light sour cream
2 tablespoons white wine
 (don't use cooking wine!)

½ teaspoon Tabasco
 (or other hot sauce)
2 tablespoons lemon juice
2 tablespoons whole-grain
 mustard sauce or Dijon mustard

Method

1. Preheat oven to 450 degrees.

2. Line baking sheet with aluminum foil and season both sides of fish with salt and white pepper. Place fish on the aluminum foil.

3. In a small bowl, whisk the sour cream, white wine, Tabasco, lemon juice and mustard. Spoon 2 tablespoons of the creamy lemon-mustard sauce over each salmon filet.

4. Bake the salmon for 15 minutes (or until center is done).

Chef's Notes

Serve with sides of whole-grain pilaf and spinach sautéed in extra-virgin olive oil and garlic. Try some of the other tasty and more exotic whole grains such as quinoa or amaranth. If you don't have time for pilaf, try a side dish of corn (save time and use frozen corn kernels). If using frozen corn kernels, heat in the microwave *without* water.

Sautéed Chicken Breasts with Basil & Cheese

SERVES 4

3 GRAMS SATURATED FAT PER SERVING

Ingredients

1¼ pounds boneless, skinless,
thin-cutlet, chicken breasts
White pepper, to taste
Salt, to taste
1 tablespoon extra-virgin olive oil
4 garlic cloves, finely chopped
Approximately 20 fresh basil leaves

4 ounces lean ham (sliced medium-thick)
¼ cup goat cheese (or substitute
light feta cheese)
Whole-wheat flour, for dusting chicken
1½ cups white wine
(do not use cooking wine)

Method

1. Season both sides of chicken with white pepper and salt.

2. Heat a nonstick or cast-iron skillet over medium heat. Add the olive oil. When oil is hot, toss in garlic and basil and cook for about 2 minutes. Transfer basil and garlic to a plate. Do not wash the skillet.

3. Lay chicken on flat surface. On one half of each piece of chicken, place a slice of ham, followed by 1 tablespoon of the goat cheese, plus a dollop of the garlic-basil mixture (save some of the garlic-basil mixture for later). Fold the chicken over and pinch the edges with your fingertips to form a "package."

4. Reheat the "dirty" skillet and throw in a bit of salt. Dust chicken packages lightly with flour. Brown chicken for about 4 minutes on each side (chicken should turn a lovely golden-brown and be done in the middle). Transfer browned chicken to a plate.

5. Raise the heat of the skillet and pour in the wine; bring the wine to a boil. Pour the wine over the chicken and top with a bit of the reserved garlic-basil mixture and serve.

Chef's Notes

This is a twist on a classic Roman dish. We love to pair chicken with whole-grain barley and green beans. Season the barley with minced garlic sautéed in extra-virgin olive oil plus a dash of salt and white pepper.

Seared Tofu with Turmeric Red Pepper Curry

SERVES 4

1.5 GRAMS SATURATED FAT PER SERVING

Ingredients

One 12-ounce jar roasted red peppers, drained well and patted dry with a paper towel (or 5 freshly roasted and peeled red peppers)

2 tablespoons Neufchatel cream cheese (or whipped cream cheese)

2 teaspoons turmeric plus extra to taste

2 packages extra-firm tofu (30 ounces total)

Salt, to taste

White pepper, to taste

2 teaspoons extra-virgin olive oil

Method

1. Toss the roasted red peppers, cream cheese and measured turmeric into a blender and blend until smooth and creamy.

2. Drain tofu and blot dry with paper towels (use several paper towels in order to get the tofu as dry as possible). Cut tofu into ¾-inch cubes and set on paper towels or a terry cloth towel, then blot gently again with more paper towels. Season all sides of the tofu with turmeric, salt and white pepper.

3. Heat the olive oil in a large nonstick skillet over medium-high heat. When the skillet is hot, add the tofu and lightly brown on each side, stirring occasionally (cook about 3 to 4 minutes a side).

4. Add the red pepper curry sauce to the tofu and continue cooking for several minutes (toss tofu gently in the sauce several times).

5. Serve warm.

Chef's Notes

Warming and lightly aromatic, this tofu recipe has East Indian flair. The turmeric is flavorful yet not overpowering, and the Neufchatel cream cheese provides a wonderful richness to the curry sauce with only a smidgen of added saturated fat. Serve with sides of petite peas and quinoa.

South of the Border Chili-Studded Meatloaf

SERVES 8

5 GRAMS SATURATED FAT PER SERVING

Ingredients

Olive oil cooking spray
1 Spanish onion, finely chopped
½ cup carrots, shredded
  (buy preshredded carrots
  to save time)
1 red bell pepper, finely chopped
1 cup frozen corn, thawed
1 can (4.5 ounces) chopped green
  chilies (found in the ethnic section
  of your supermarket)
½ cup fresh cilantro, chopped
1 pound extra-lean ground beef
  (10 percent or less fat)

2 eggs
2 cups fresh salsa, divided
  (in the deli section of
  your supermarket)
¾ cup wheat germ
¾ cup low-fat mozzarella
  cheese, shredded
1 tablespoon cumin
1 teaspoon chili powder
1 teaspoon salt

Method

1. Preheat the oven to 350 degrees and spray a rectangular 10-x-14-inch casserole dish with olive oil cooking spray.

2. In a large bowl, mix with your hands the vegetables (onion, carrots, bell pepper, corn, canned chilies) and cilantro, then mix in the ground beef and eggs. Add 1 cup of salsa and the wheat germ, cheese, cumin, chili powder and salt.

3. Shape the meat mixture into a loaf and place in the center of the casserole; pat and shape the loaf with your hands.

4. Bake the meatloaf for 30 minutes, then baste with the remaining 1 cup of salsa. Bake for another 40 to 45 minutes until cooked through. Let stand 15 minutes before slicing.

Chef's Notes

Mexican food lovers will go crazy for this flavor-packed twist on a classic standby.

Spiced Pork Chops with Apple Onion Compote

SERVES 4

3.5 GRAMS SATURATED FAT PER SERVING

Ingredients

4 boneless center-cut pork loin chops
(about 1 pound total) meticulously
trimmed of all fat and
pounded thin (see directions below)

2 teaspoons dried basil

2 teaspoons paprika

½ teaspoon salt, plus more to taste

1 teaspoon ground black pepper

4 teaspoons extra-virgin olive oil

2 large Spanish onions, thinly
sliced into rounds

2 tablespoons apple cider vinegar

⅓ cup apple juice

2 large Granny Smith apples, peeled,
cored and cut into wedges

1 cup all-natural chicken broth

¼ cup whole milk

Method

1. Place pork chops in a ziplock bag and pound thin.

2. In a small bowl, mix the dried basil, paprika, measured salt and pepper. Rub the spice mixture onto both sides of the pork chops and set aside.

3. In a large, deep, nonstick frying pan heat 3 teaspoons extra-virgin olive oil over medium-high heat. Add the onion and sauté until lightly browned, approximately 5 minutes. Transfer the onion to a large plate.

4. Add the remaining teaspoon of olive oil to the "dirty" skillet and reheat it over medium-high heat. Add the pork chops and sear until lightly browned on both sides (3 to 4 minutes each side). Put the pork on the plate with the onion.

5. Return the pan to medium heat and pour in the vinegar and apple juice. Using a spatula, scrape the browned bits from the bottom of the pan. Return the pork chops and the onion to the pan and set the apple wedges on top of the pork. Pour in the chicken broth, cover and simmer (reduce the heat if the liquid begins to boil); simmer until the pork chops are cooked throughout, about 12 to 15 minutes.

6. Transfer the chops, apple wedges and onion to individual serving plates. Pour the milk into the pan, raise the heat to high and boil for about 5 to 6 minutes. Pour the sauce over the pork chops and serve at once.

Stir-Fried Chicken with Pecans and Mushrooms

SERVES 4

1.5 GRAMS SATURATED FAT PER SERVING

Ingredients

1 pound skinless, boneless
chicken breasts

3-inch piece fresh gingerroot,
peeled and thinly sliced

3 tablespoons soy sauce

1 tablespoon brown sugar

1 tablespoon high-oleic canola oil

1 pound fresh button
mushrooms, halved

½ cup chopped pecans

2 teaspoons honey

Coarse black pepper

Method

1. Cut the chicken into thin strips and place in a bowl. Add the thinly sliced ginger, soy sauce and brown sugar. Mix well, cover and let marinate for at least 1 hour.

2. Heat the canola oil over medium-high heat in a wok or large frying pan. Add the chicken and cook 4 to 5 minutes, stirring constantly.

3. Turn the heat to high, add the mushrooms and pecans, and cook, stirring constantly, until the chicken is cooked through and vegetables are tender but still crisp.

4. Stir in the honey, season with pepper and serve at once.

Chef's Notes

Serve this Asian-inspired dish over a small mound of brown rice with a side of steamed asparagus.

Sun-Dried Tomato Mozzarella Chicken

SERVES 4

3 GRAMS SATURATED FAT PER SERVING

Ingredients

1¼ pounds of boneless, skinless, thin-cutlet chicken breasts

White pepper, to taste

Parsley flakes, for seasoning

2 teaspoons extra-virgin olive oil

½ cup sun-dried tomatoes, chopped

½ cup black olives, sliced thin

White wine

½ lemon, juice only

½ cup low-fat mozzarella, shredded

Method

1. Season both sides of chicken breasts with pepper and parsley flakes.

2. Heat 2 teaspoons olive oil in a heavy skillet over medium-high heat. When hot, sear chicken breasts on one side for 2 minutes.

3. Flip chicken breasts and add sun-dried tomatoes and olives. Sear the other side of the chicken for another 2 minutes.

4. Add enough wine to the skillet to just barely cover the chicken breasts. Cover and cook for 5 to 6 minutes. Add lemon juice and cook for an additional minute (or until chicken is done).

5. Top each chicken breast with the mozzarella cheese, cover with a lid for 1 additional minute (or until cheese is melted). Serve warm.

Chef's Notes

Enhance this Mediterranean-style dish with a side of whole-wheat couscous and roasted asparagus. To roast the asparagus, mix asparagus with a bit of extra-virgin olive oil, salt and white pepper, then place in a tin-foil-lined baking dish and roast uncovered at 450 degrees for 15 minutes.

Veggie-Lovers Lasagna

SERVES 9

3.5 GRAMS SATURATED FAT PER SERVING

Ingredients

1 package (14 ounces) extra-firm tofu

1 tablespoon extra-virgin olive oil

4 to 5 garlic cloves, chopped

3½ cups carrots, shredded (save time and buy preshredded carrots)

1 cup fresh basil, chopped

¼ teaspoon white pepper, plus more to taste

1 cup large curd cottage cheese (use full-fat rather than low-fat)

1 small package (10 ounces) frozen chopped spinach, thawed and thoroughly drained and patted dry with paper towels

½ cup Parmesan cheese

½ teaspoon salt, plus more to taste

1 tablespoon dried oregano

Two 25-ounce jars (50 total ounces) of high-quality prepared marinara sauce (I like Rao's Marinara Joey Pots and Pans Marinara, or Emeril's Roasted Red Pepper)

10 ounces (12 total noodles) raw whole-wheat lasagna noodles (the noodles will cook while the lasagna bakes)

1 cup low-fat mozzarella cheese, shredded

Method

1. Tofu prep: Thoroughly drain all excess water from the tofu, then thoroughly pat dry with either a terry cloth towel or paper towels. Crumble tofu and pat dry again.

2. Preheat the oven to 350 degrees.

3. Heat 1 tablespoon extra-virgin olive oil in a skillet over medium heat and sauté garlic and carrots for 3 to 4 minutes. Add the fresh basil and a dash of white pepper; stir gently until basil wilts. Remove from heat.

4. In a large bowl, mix the tofu, cottage cheese, spinach, Parmesan cheese, ½ teaspoon salt, ¼ teaspoon white pepper and oregano.

5. Spread 1 cup of sauce on the bottom of an extra large 15-x-10-inch casserole dish. (**Note:** *the lasagna will only take up ¾ of the casserole dish but it is important to use an extra large dish so that liquid from the vegetables can drain onto one side.*) Arrange 4 lasagna noodles on top of the sauce and then add 1 cup of sauce on top of the noodles. Spread half of the cottage cheese, tofu and spinach mixture on top of the sauce.

6. Add 1 more cup of sauce, another layer of noodles, and another cup of

sauce. Spread all of the carrot and basil mixture on top of the sauce, and then add the remaining half of the cottage cheese, tofu and spinach mixture.

7. Top with 1 cup of sauce, another layer of noodles and another cup of sauce. Top with the shredded mozzarella cheese, cover loosely with tin foil and bake for 55 minutes.

8. When done, let sit in the oven for 20 to 25 minutes before serving. Serve warm.

Chef's Notes

Nothing beats the comfort of delicious lasagna. Be sure to choose a high-quality marinara sauce when making this recipe (or any recipe for that matter!). Although lasagna may seem intimidating, it really is rather easy to prepare. And of course it can be made well in advance. If you don't have a large family, this recipe can be served for at least two nights and possibly three; simply cover tightly and store in the refrigerator. To stretch out the meal, add a fresh side salad of spinach with a simple vinaigrette dressing.

15 Veggies with Flair

Bistro-Style Oven-Roasted Veggies & Potatoes

SERVES 6

0 GRAMS SATURATED FAT PER SERVING

Ingredients

5 medium red-skinned potatoes

2 red bell peppers, chopped into
bite-size pieces

2 zucchini, chopped into ½-inch chunks

2 carrots, chopped into bite-size pieces

1 small eggplant, chopped into
bite-size pieces

1 red onion, cut into bite-size pieces

6 to 10 cloves garlic, coarsely chopped

3 tablespoons fresh chopped rosemary

Salt and white pepper to taste

¼ cup extra-virgin olive oil

Method

1. Wash potatoes and place them in a medium-size pot. Cover with water and simmer until the potatoes are just fork tender (about 20 minutes). Cut the potatoes into ½-inch cubes.

2. Preheat oven to 450 degrees.

3. Place all of the vegetables in a bowl and toss with the olive oil, garlic, rosemary, salt and white pepper.

4. Line two cookie sheets with tin foil and spread the vegetables in a single layer on the sheets. Roast the vegetables in the oven for 20 minutes (or until almost tender).

5. Broil for 8 to 10 minutes, or until the edges of the vegetables are brown.

Chef's Notes

The fresh rosemary is what gives this down-home recipe its gourmet touch.

Butternut Squash Soufflé

SERVES 6

2.5 GRAMS SATURATED FAT PER SERVING

Ingredients

Canola oil cooking spray
1 tablespoon butter
3 tablespoons whole-wheat flour
1 cup 2% milk
1¼ cup cooked pureed butternut
squash or one package (12 ounces)
Birds Eye Cooked Winter Squash

¼ teaspoon nutmeg
¼ teaspoon salt
¼ teaspoon white pepper
¼ cup Splenda sugar substitute
4 eggs, separated

Method

1. Preheat the oven to 350 degrees and spray the bottom and sides of a 1½-quart casserole or soufflé dish with canola oil cooking spray.

2. In a large nonstick skillet, heat the butter over low heat. When the butter melts, add the flour and mix quickly and thoroughly with a fork. Continue stirring the flour and gradually add the milk. Cook over low heat for 5 to 6 minutes, stirring frequently, until the sauce is thick and smooth.

3. Mix the squash with the sauce and season with nutmeg, salt, white pepper and Splenda. Remove from heat.

4. Use an electric mixer and beat the egg yolks until light; then add 3 tablespoons of the butternut squash sauce to the egg yolks. Add the egg yolk mixture to the sauce, blend well, and transfer to the prepared casserole or soufflé dish.

5. Use an electric mixer and beat the egg whites until stiff, not dry. Gently and thoroughly fold the egg white mixture in with the squash mixture. Bake for 35 minutes at 350 degrees until firm, puffed and lightly browned. Serve immediately.

Chef's Notes

A soufflé always makes a striking presentation. Serve with simple sides of grilled or broiled fish, corn on the cob and whole-grain bread.

Chilled Balsamic Broccoli

SERVES 4

0 GRAMS SATURATED FAT PER SERVING

Ingredients

1 head fresh broccoli, cut into
  bite-size pieces (including the stems)
5 to 6 cloves
  garlic, coarsely chopped
¼ cup balsamic vinegar
1 tablespoon flaxseed oil
  (we recommend Barlean's brand)

1 tablespoon extra-virgin olive oil
Dried oregano, to taste
Salt
Coarsely ground black pepper

Method

1. Fill a large bowl with ice and water.

2. Bring several inches of water to a boil in a large covered pot. Add the broccoli and garlic to the boiling water, cover and cook for 3 to 4 minutes (or until just tender when pierced with a fork) and immediately drain. Do not overcook; broccoli should be firm-tender. Immediately plunge the broccoli and garlic into the ice water bath for 2 minutes.

3. Drain broccoli and garlic again and place in a gallon-size ziplock bag.

4. To the ziplock bag add balsamic vinegar, oils, oregano, salt and pepper.

5. Chill the broccoli-filled ziplock bag in the freezer for 10–15 minutes or in refrigerator for 30 minutes until cold. Serve cold.

Chef's Notes

This is a snap to make when you are in a hurry and need a healthy and delicious-tasting vegetable side dish.

Gourmet-Lovers Broccoli and Cheese Casserole

SERVES 6

2.5 GRAMS SATURATED FAT PER SERVING

Ingredients

Olive oil cooking spray

¾ cup whole-wheat bread crumbs, divided (see Chef's Notes)

¾ pound broccoli, cut into 1-inch pieces

2 tablespoons extra-virgin olive oil

1 cup 2% milk

2 large shallots, finely diced

¼ cup low-fat Swiss cheese, grated

¼ cup Parmesan cheese, grated

2 eggs, separated

½ teaspoon salt, or to taste

½ teaspoon white pepper, or to taste

Method

1. Preheat the oven to 375 degrees. Spray the bottom and sides of an 8-x-10-inch casserole dish with nonstick cooking spray. Sprinkle one-quarter cup of whole-wheat bread crumbs on the bottom of the dish.

2. Steam the broccoli until barely tender when pierced with a knife and then drain, rinse and chop finely. Pat the broccoli with paper towels to dry thoroughly.

3. In a medium nonstick skillet, heat 1 tablespoon extra-virgin olive oil over medium heat; when the oil is hot, add the remaining bread crumbs and brown lightly. Then stir in the milk (don't worry if the mixture looks a little odd). When the milk and bread crumbs are hot, transfer the mixture to large bowl.

4. Heat the remaining 1 tablespoon of extra-virgin olive oil in the "dirty" skillet over medium-heat and then sauté the shallots until translucent (about 3 minutes). Remove shallots from heat and transfer to the bowl with the bread crumb mixture.

5. Add the broccoli, two cheeses and egg yolks to the bowl with the bread crumbs and shallots. Season with salt and white pepper. Transfer the mixture to the prepared casserole dish.

6. Beat the egg whites until stiff then fold them into the broccoli and cheese mixture. Bake at 375 degrees for 25 minutes or until puffed and browned. Serve immediately.

Chef's Notes

You can either buy whole-wheat bread crumbs at a natural foods store or make your own. To make your own, pulse 2 to 3 toasted whole-wheat toast slices in a food processor with a teaspoon of extra-virgin olive oil and a pinch of salt.

Lemon-Splashed Braised Red Cabbage

SERVES 4

2 GRAMS SATURATED FAT PER SERVING

Ingredients

1 teaspoon butter

2 teaspoons extra-virgin olive oil

6 cups shredded red cabbage
  (buy preshredded bagged red cabbage)

Juice from ½ whole lemon

Salt and white pepper to taste

Method

1. Melt butter with the extra-virgin olive oil in a large skillet over medium heat. Add cabbage and toss to coat.

2. Add the juice from the lemon and toss lemon half into the skillet; mix cabbage with a spoon, cover, and simmer for 5 minutes.

3. Uncover and continue to simmer and stir until cabbage is soft but not mushy. Season to taste with salt and white pepper.

Chef's Notes

Save time and purchase prebagged, prewashed vegetables when available.

Luscious Leeks with Lemon

SERVES 4

0 GRAMS SATURATED FAT PER SERVING

Ingredients

1 pound leeks, cleaned and cut
(see cleaning tips below)
1 tablespoon extra-virgin olive oil
3 to 4 cloves garlic, chopped

1 whole lemon, sliced in half and deseeded
1 small can sliced mushrooms
Salt, to taste
White pepper, to taste

Method

1. Leeks must be washed meticulously. Begin by cutting off the root and cutting the leeks into 2-inch pieces. Spray each leaf with water to remove any and all traces of dirt.

2. Heat olive oil in a large pot over medium-high heat.

3. When oil is hot, add chopped garlic and sauté briefly (careful not to brown the garlic).

4. Add cut leeks and mix with a large spoon to coat leaves in oil. Squeeze the juice of a whole lemon into the pot of leeks, then drop the lemon halves into the pot. Add the mushrooms, toss gently and cover.

5. Lower the heat and cook leeks about 5 minutes, stirring several times during cooking process. Leeks will be firm-soft when done.

6. Season with salt and white pepper to taste and serve warm.

Chef's Notes

Never tried leeks? This is one of our favorite standby vegetable recipes, and we hope you experiment; you won't be disappointed. Leeks always get rave reviews from our dinner guests.

Parmesan Asparagus Roast

SERVES 6
2 GRAMS SATURATED FAT PER SERVING

Ingredients

3 pounds fresh asparagus spears,
  washed and trimmed (snap off tough ends)
1 tablespoon dry white wine
1 tablespoon extra-virgin olive oil

Salt and white pepper
Lemon juice from ½ lemon
¼ cup whole *shaved* Parmesan cheese

Method

1. Preheat the oven to 450 degrees.

2. Toss asparagus spears with the wine and extra-virgin olive oil.

3. Line a cookie sheet with aluminum foil and arrange asparagus spears on top. Sprinkle asparagus with salt and white pepper.

4. Roast asparagus for approximately 8 minutes, depending on the thickness of the spears, until crisp-tender. Remove asparagus from the oven and drizzle with lemon juice and top with shaved Parmesan.

5. Return asparagus to the oven and roast for 1 to 2 minutes longer.

Chef's Notes

If you snap the tough ends from the asparagus, as opposed to cutting them, you will be sure to remove all of the tough bottom portions (not every asparagus spear is tender at the same point). If you want the spears perfectly uniform for visual appeal, just snap first, then cut to make them equal in size.

Roasted Beets with Goat Cheese

SERVES 4

1 GRAM SATURATED FAT PER SERVING

Ingredients

2 bunches fresh beets
(about 5 medium-size beet bulbs),
washed, trimmed and greens chopped
into bite-size pieces
1 tablespoon extra-virgin olive oil, divided

2 teaspoons sugar
2 teaspoons balsamic vinegar
Juice from ½ lemon
¼ teaspoon salt
2 tablespoons goat cheese

Method

1. Preheat oven to 400 degrees.

2. Wrap whole beet bulbs individually in aluminum foil and roast in the oven for about 30 to 40 minutes or until tender when pierced with a fork.

3. Meanwhile, sauté the beet greens in a skillet over medium-high heat with 2 teaspoons of extra-virgin olive oil until just wilted. Remove from heat and transfer the greens to a large bowl.

4. When beet bulbs are done, cut into wedges and place in the bowl with the beet greens.

5. In a small bowl make the vinaigrette by mixing the sugar, vinegar, lemon juice, salt and remaining teaspoon of the extra-virgin olive oil. Gently toss the vinaigrette in with the beets and beet greens. Top with dollops of goat cheese. Serve at once.

Chef's Notes

Chances are you have never tried fresh beets. We promise that fresh and properly prepared beets taste absolutely nothing like the canned stuff you may have tried and detested in the past. This beet dish is delicious!

16 "In Vogue" Starches

BASIC BEAN PREPARATION

To soften by soaking, place beans in a large pot and fill the pot with water; cover and let beans sit for the recommended soak time. Cooked beans can be stored in a covered container in the refrigerator for up to 4 days. Having prepared beans handy will allow you to quickly incorporate these nutritious foods into your meals with ease. **Note:** *Avoid cooking beans in salted water because they'll become tough; instead, salt the beans after they've been cooked.*

1 Cup Beans	Soak Time	Water + Cook Time (on high heat)
Adzuki	————————-	4 cups water + 1½ hours
Black Beans	4 hours	3 cups water + 1½ hours
Black-eyed Peas	————————-	4 cups water + 1 hour
Chickpeas	Overnight (6 to 8 hours)	3 cups water + 1½ hours
Great Northern	Overnight (6 to 8 hours)	3 cups water + 1½ hours
Kidney	Overnight (6 to 8 hours)	3 cups water + 1½ hours
Lentils	————————	4 cups water + 20-40 minutes
Navy	Overnight (6 to 8 hours)	3 cups water + 1½ hours
Soybeans	Overnight (6 to 8 hours)	3 cups water + 1½ hours
Green or Yellow Split Peas	————————	4 cups water + 45 minutes

Note: To speed up and ease bean preparation, invest in a good quality pressure cooker; pressure-cooked beans cook in a fraction of the time.

BASIC GRAIN PREPARATION

Cooked grains are excellent eaten as a side dish or added to soups, salads and pilafs. Make grains ahead and store in a covered container in the refrigerator for 2 to 3 days. Be sure to rinse grains before cooking to eliminate any bitterness. To cook grains quickly, add a little bit of salt, cover with a lid and cook on high heat.

1 Cup Grain	Water + Cook Time (on high heat)
Amaranth	2½ cups water + 20 to 25 minutes
Barley, whole	3 cups water + 1 hour
Buckwheat	3 cups water + 20 minutes
Bulgar	2 cups water + 20 minutes
Corn, grits	3 cups water + 15 minutes
Kamut	3 cups water + 1½ hours
Millet	3 cups water + 25 minutes
Oats, steel cut	3 cups water + 8 minutes
Quinoa	2 cups water + 15 to 20 minutes
Rice, basmati, brown	2 cups water + 40 minutes
Rice, brown, long and short grain	2 cups water + 45 minutes
Rye	3 cups water + 50 to 60 minutes
Spelt	3 cups water + 60 minutes
Triticale	3 cups water + 60 minutes
Wheat berries	4 cups water + 45 to 60 minutes
Wild rice	2½ cups + 60 minutes

Note: For ease of preparation, invest in a high-quality rice cooker with an automatic timer. When cooking with a rice cooker simply measure your grain and water, set the timer and let it cook—no pot watching.

Apple & Ginger–Spiked Sweet Potato Casserole

SERVES 6

1.25 GRAMS SATURATED FAT PER SERVING

Ingredients

Canola oil cooking spray

2 Granny Smith apples, peeled,
cored and sliced into rounds

2 large sweet potatoes, peeled and
sliced into rounds

¼ cup pickled ginger (in the sushi section
of your supermarket), rinsed,
patted dry and chopped

½ teaspoon salt

3 tablespoons fresh lemon juice

½ cup water, less 2 tablespoons

3 tablespoons honey

1 tablespoon butter, melted

Method

1. Preheat the oven to 375 degrees and spray an 8-inch-square baking dish with cooking spray. Arrange half of the apple rounds in the baking dish; top with half of the sliced sweet potatoes. Sprinkle with half of the ginger and half of the salt and repeat the layers.

2. In a small bowl, mix the lemon juice, water and honey. Pour the liquid over the sweet potatoes. Cover with aluminum foil and bake for 45 minutes; remove from the oven and pour the melted butter evenly on top of the sweet potatoes and bake for an additional 15 minutes, or until lightly browned.

3. Allow to cool and serve at once.

Chef's Notes

Not your ordinary sweet potato casserole, our version adds much more flavor and zip than the standard (and not so healthy) marshmallow mess.

Mexicali Black Bean & Corn Salsa

SERVES 8

3 GRAMS SATURATED FAT PER SERVING

Ingredients

Vinaigrette:

2 teaspoons brown sugar

2 to 3 cloves garlic, crushed

1 tablespoon apple cider vinegar

2 tablespoons lime juice

2 tablespoons flaxseed oil
  (we recommend Barlean's brand)

2 tablespoons extra-virgin olive oil

Salsa:

1 large can (1 pound, 13 ounces) of
  black beans, well-rinsed and drained

3 cups frozen yellow corn kernels,
  thawed (do not cook!)

1 red bell peppers, finely chopped

½ cup scallions, finely chopped

½ small red onion, finely chopped

½ cup parsley, chopped

1 tablespoon cumin

¼ teaspoon salt

4 ounces fresh buffalo mozzarella,
  thinly sliced

Method

Vinaigrette:

In a small bowl, combine all of the ingredients for the vinaigrette and whisk well.

Salsa:

1. In a large bowl, combine the first 6 ingredients for the salsa; mix well. Add the cumin and salt and toss gently to combine. Fold in the vinaigrette, top with fresh slices of buffalo mozzarella, cover and refrigerate.

2. Serve cold.

Chef's Notes

Quick and easy to prepare, this Mexican-inspired salsa is perfect for serving at an outdoor barbecue. As an alternative to the cheese, this salsa is also delicious served with fresh sliced avocado (if you swap avocado for cheese, the recipe will contain 0 grams of saturated fat). If you choose to use the avocado instead of the cheese, wait until serving time to slice the avocado; otherwise the avocado will turn colors. Keep the salsa refrigerated and serve cold to keep the flaxseed oil fresh.

Parsley & Horseradish Mashed Red Potatoes

SERVES 6

1 GRAM SATURATED FAT PER SERVING

Ingredients

8 medium-size red potatoes
   (about 2 pounds)
2 tablespoons extra-virgin olive oil
¼ cup prepared fresh horseradish
¼ cup light cream

Salt, to taste
Black pepper, to taste
1 cup loosely packed fresh
   parsley, finely chopped

Method

1. Bring a large pot of salted water to a boil. Boil potatoes for 28 to 30 minutes or until easily pierced with a fork. Meanwhile, in a small bowl, mix the extra-virgin olive oil, horseradish and light cream.

2. Drain potatoes when done and transfer to a large cookie sheet. Cut the potatoes into small pieces with two knives, then mash with a potato masher.

3. Transfer the potatoes to a large bowl and mash in the horseradish mixture. Continue mashing with a potato masher (you may also use a handheld electric blender) until all ingredients are well combined.

4. Season to taste with salt and pepper. Mix in the parsley and serve warm.

Chef's Notes

We always recommend leaving the skins on your potatoes whenever possible. By doing so you'll reap three benefits: (1) the dish will be easier and quicker to prepare, (2) you'll get more fiber and (3) you'll get more flavor.

Penne Pasta with Tomato Basil Cream Sauce

SERVES 4

2 GRAMS SATURATED FAT PER SERVING

Ingredients

1 tablespoon plus 1 teaspoon
extra-virgin olive oil

1 heaping tablespoon minced
garlic cloves

4 fresh and firm medium-size
tomatoes (such as Holland
Beefsteak variety), peeled, seeded
and chopped

½ cup dry white wine
(do not use cooking wine)

1 cup loosely packed fresh basil
leaves, chopped

¼ cup light cream

Salt, to taste

White pepper, to taste

4 cups whole-wheat penne pasta,
cooked al dente

2 tablespoons Parmesan cheese

Method

1. Heat the extra-virgin olive oil in a large nonstick skillet over medium heat. Add the garlic and gently sauté for 1 minute.

2. Raise the heat to medium-high and add the tomatoes, wine and basil. Simmer for 12 minutes, stirring occasionally. Pour in the cream and simmer for another 2 to 3 minutes. Season to taste with salt and white pepper.

3. Mix in the penne and Parmesan and serve warm.

Chef's Notes

Even if tomatoes are not your thing, you'll still love this recipe. It's rich, creamy and simply delicious.

Quinoa & Cashew–Stuffed Peppers

SERVES 8

1.5 GRAMS SATURATED FAT PER SERVING

Ingredients

1 cup *uncooked* quinoa
2 cups all-natural chicken broth
4 medium red bell peppers,
  halved lengthwise and deseeded
1 tablespoon extra-virgin olive oil
3 cloves garlic, minced
½ Spanish onion, finely diced

1 cup shredded carrots
½ cup whole cashews, finely chopped
1 teaspoon chili powder
Tabasco or other hot sauce, to taste
1 cup *fresh* cilantro, washed and finely chopped
1 cup low-fat shredded mozzarella cheese

Method

1. Preheat the oven to 350 degrees.

2. Place quinoa and chicken broth in a large saucepan and bring to a boil. Reduce to a simmer, cover and cook, stirring occasionally, until the liquid is absorbed (about 15 minutes). Set aside. **Note:** *Quinoa may be cooked and stored in the refrigerator for up to 2 days before stuffing the peppers.*

3. Soften the red peppers by placing them in a pot of boiling water for several minutes; remove the peppers when they are soft, but do not allow them to get limp.

4. Heat the olive oil in a skillet over medium heat. Sauté the garlic, onion and carrots until the onions are soft. Add the cashews and sauté for a minute longer. Fold in the quinoa and gently stir. Season the mixture with chili powder and a dash of hot sauce. Stir in the cilantro. Turn off the heat and set mixture aside.

6. Line a baking pan with aluminum foil; place peppers on the foil and fill with the quinoa mixture. Top each pepper with shredded mozzarella cheese.

7. Bake for 30 minutes.

Chef's Notes

These stuffed peppers make an exciting-looking and tasty side dish. Serve with a simple fresh spinach salad and grilled fish.

Santa Fe-Style Baked Mac & Cheese

SERVES 6

4.75 GRAMS SATURATED FAT PER SERVING

Ingredients

1 can (7 ounces) chipotle peppers in adobo sauce (such as La Costena brand, found in the Latin foods section of your local supermarket). **Note:** *This brand does contain safflower oil, but less than ½ gram per serving. Because you will only be using a smidgen, this product is acceptable.*

1 tablespoon extra-virgin olive oil

1 can (4.5 ounces) chopped green chiles (such as Old El Paso brand, also found in the Latin foods section of your local supermarket)

1 cup finely chopped onion

1 cup finely chopped green bell pepper

2 garlic cloves, minced

2 tablespoons whole-wheat flour

1 (14½ ounce) can diced tomatoes, drained

4 cups cooked whole-wheat elbow macaroni

1½ cups low-fat sharp cheddar cheese

1 cup 1% low-fat cottage cheese

1 cup 1% reduced-fat milk

¼ cup Parmesan cheese

1 large egg, lightly beaten

Cooking spray

¼ cup wheat germ

Method

1. Preheat the oven to 350 degrees.

2. Remove 2 chipotle peppers from the can and finely chop. Remove 1 teaspoon of the adobo sauce from the can and set aside. (If you want a less spicy dish do not add the teaspoon of adobo sauce.) Save the remaining can of chipotle peppers for another time.

3. In a large heavy skillet heat the oil over medium-high heat. Add the chipotle peppers, the chopped green chiles, onion, bell pepper and garlic. Sauté for about 5 minutes or until onion is soft, stirring frequently. Sprinkle flour on top of the mixture and stir constantly for 1 minute.

4. Mix in the tomatoes and reduce the heat to medium. Cook for 3 to 4 minutes or until sauce thickens. Add the reserved teaspoon of adobo sauce, cooked macaroni, cheddar cheese, cottage cheese, milk, Parmesan and egg. Stir to combine.

5. Spoon the macaroni mixture into a 2-quart baking dish coated with

cooking spray; top with wheat germ. Bake for 40 minutes. Remove from oven and allow the macaroni and cheese to sit for at least 10 minutes before serving.

Chef's Notes

This grown-up-style macaroni and cheese dish can stand alone as an entrée. Serve with a side salad of mixed greens.

Savory Black & White Bean Puree

SERVES 8

0 GRAMS SATURATED FAT PER SERVING

Ingredients

1 tablespoon extra-virgin olive oil

1 Spanish onion, chopped

1 green or red pepper, chopped

3 cloves garlic, chopped

2 (15-ounce) cans black beans, rinsed and drained

1 (15-ounce) can cannelloni beans, rinsed and drained

1 cup chicken broth (optional)

3 cups water

2 tablespoons red wine, optional (don't use cooking wine!)

1 teaspoon cumin

1 teaspoon Tabasco (or other hot sauce)

Salt, to taste

Freshly ground black pepper, to taste

Low-fat sour cream, for garnish

Method

1. In a large soup pot heat the extra-virgin olive oil over medium heat and sauté the onion, pepper and garlic until tender.

2. In a food processor or blender, puree the black beans, cannelloni beans, chicken broth and water (this will have to be done in several batches).

3. Transfer the pureed beans to the soup pot and add the red wine, cumin, Tabasco, salt and freshly ground black pepper. Mix and gently simmer for 30 minutes.

4. Serve warm and garnish with a dollop of sour cream.

Chef's Notes

No need to slave away all day preparing time-consuming beans from scratch. Even the best chefs use canned beans; the secret is to wash and drain the beans thoroughly. Keeping several cans of beans on the pantry shelf is a rescue staple when you're crunched for time but still want to prepare a healthy meal.

Spicy Bahamian Black Bean Fritters

SERVES 9

1 GRAM SATURATED FAT PER SERVING

Ingredients

1 (28-ounce) can black beans (rinsed and drained)

1 teaspoon ground cumin

2 teaspoons chili powder

½ cup spicy jalapeño cheese, shredded

½ cup carrots, shredded (buy preshredded carrots to save time)

¼ cup wheat germ

½ cup fresh cilantro, chopped

¼ teaspoon salt (or more to taste)

1 tablespoon lime juice

2 teaspoons Tabasco sauce

Whole-wheat flour for dusting

Cornmeal (stone-ground) for dusting

2 tablespoons extra-virgin olive oil

Reduced-fat sour cream, for garnish

Salsa, for garnish

Method

1. Roughly mash the beans in a large bowl, then add the cumin, chili powder, shredded cheese, shredded carrots, wheat germ, cilantro, salt, lime juice and Tabasco.

2. Refrigerate the bean mixture for 20 minutes. Form into ½-inch cakes (about 3 inches across).

3. Lightly dust both sides of the bean cakes with whole wheat flour and place on wax paper; return bean cakes to the refrigerator for 10 minutes.

4. Remove the bean cakes from the refrigerator and dust both sides with cornmeal.

5. Heat 1 tablespoon extra-virgin olive in a large skillet over medium heat and cook half of the bean cakes for 3 to 4 minutes on each side (or until they form a crust).

6. Repeat step 5 with the second batch of bean cakes.

7. Serve bean cakes with a spoonful of reduced-fat sour cream and salsa.

Chef's Notes

Serve these yummy and fiber-rich bean fritters as an appetizer or as a side dish to grilled chicken or fish.

Summer Spelt Salad

SERVES 6

0 GRAMS SATURATED FAT PER SERVING

Ingredients

2 cups cooked spelt (see basic grain preparation guide on page 333)

2 yellow bell peppers, finely chopped

¼ cup chopped parsley

1 tablespoon canola oil mayonnaise

1 tablespoon flaxseed oil (we recommend Barlean's brand)

2 tablespoons lemon juice

2 teaspoons brown sugar

Salt, to taste

Method

1. In a large bowl, combine the spelt, bell peppers and parsley.

2. In a small bowl, whisk the mayonnaise, flaxseed oil and lemon juice. Add the brown sugar and mix well.

3. Pour the dressing over the spelt and toss to combine. Season with salt to taste. Cover and chill for one hour before serving.

Chef's Notes

This summer salad is refreshing and simple to make. If you're new to spelt, you'll be pleasantly surprised with its unique and nutty flavor.

Wheat Berry Brunch Salad

SERVES 10

0 GRAMS SATURATED FAT PER SERVING

Ingredients

2 large Granny Smith apples,
  cored and chopped into
  small bite-size pieces
3 stalks celery, finely chopped
¾ cup raisins
⅓ cup lemon juice
3 tablespoons reduced-fat sour cream
1 tablespoon canola oil mayonnaise

1 packet Splenda sugar substitute
⅛ teaspoon salt
⅛ teaspoon white pepper
2 cups cooked and chilled
  and drained wheat berries (see basic grain
  preparation guide on page 333)
1 cup walnuts, finely chopped

Method

1. In a large bowl, combine the apples with the celery, then add the raisins, lemon juice, sour cream, mayonnaise, Splenda, salt and white pepper and toss gently.

2. Mix in the wheat berries and walnuts and toss gently.

3. Chill for at least 30 minutes in the refrigerator and serve cold.

Chef's Notes

As the name implies, this wheat berry salad is perfect for brunch. To form a complete meal, serve with grilled chicken and a vegetable-based soup such as butternut squash soup.

Whole-Grain Parmesan Corn Muffins

YIELDS 9 MUFFINS

0 GRAMS SATURATED FAT PER SERVING

Ingredients

Canola oil cooking spray
⅔ cup stone-ground
   whole-grain yellow cornmeal
1 cup whole-wheat flour
2 teaspoons baking powder
¼ teaspoon salt

2 tablespoons honey
⅔ cup low-fat milk
¼ cup extra-virgin olive oil
2 eggs, lightly beaten
¼ cup Parmesan cheese
1 cup frozen corn

Method

1. Preheat the oven to 425 degrees. Liberally spray muffin tins with canola oil cooking spray.

2. In a medium-size bowl, mix the cornmeal, flour, baking powder and salt. Make a well in the center of the mixture and add the honey, milk, oil, eggs and Parmesan cheese. Mix until moist. Blend in the frozen corn kernels.

3. Spoon the batter into prepared muffin tins and bake for 18 minutes or until a toothpick inserted in the middle comes out clean. Remove muffins from the muffin tins immediately and serve warm.

Chef's Notes

Serve muffins as a side dish or even for breakfast. Kids love them!

"Wild" About Rice

SERVES 8

1.5 GRAMS SATURATED FAT PER SERVING

Ingredients

1 tablespoon butter

3 cloves garlic, minced

1 small onion, chopped

2 scallions, diced

2 stalks celery, chopped

¾ cup dried apricots, chopped

¾ cup pecans, chopped

1 small can (4-ounce) mushroom stems and pieces, drained

½ cup oranges, cut into bite-size pieces

2 cups cooked wild rice (follow directions on package)

¼ cup white wine

1 teaspoon dried rosemary

½ teaspoon salt

¼ teaspoon white pepper

1 tablespoon brown sugar

Method

1. In a large nonstick pan, melt butter over medium heat. Add garlic and onions and sauté for 1 to 2 minutes.

2. Add scallions and sauté briefly. Add the celery and sauté briefly.

3. Add dried apricots and nuts and sauté 1 minute.

4. Add mushrooms and orange pieces and sauté 1 minute.

5. Add cooked wild rice and wine and sauté for an additional 3 minutes.

6. Season with rosemary, salt, white pepper and brown sugar, and toss gently. Serve warm.

Chef's Notes

Be sure to have all of your ingredients chopped and premeasured before beginning to sauté because once the cooking begins, things move fast. For variety, try substituting the wild rice for other whole grains such as wheat berries or quinoa. Wild rice also mixes well with brown rice.

Sweet Treats

Almond Apricot Bread Pudding

SERVES 10

5.5 GRAMS SATURATED FAT PER SERVING

Ingredients

1 cup slivered almonds (save time
  and buy slivered almonds)
1½ cups dried apricots, finely chopped
Canola oil cooking spray
1 cup finely chopped almonds (save time
  and buy finely chopped almonds)
7 slices whole-wheat bread, crusts removed
  (we use Alvarado Street Bakery brand
  California Style Bread)
6 eggs

½ cup packed brown sugar
7 packets Splenda brand
  all-natural sugar substitute
1 tablespoon butter, melted
½ cup mascarpone cheese, divided
1 cup soy milk
1½ teaspoons almond extract,
  plus ½ teaspoon
¼ cup low-fat sour cream
½ cup apricot jelly

Method

1. Preheat the oven to 375 degrees.

2. In a medium-size bowl, combine the slivered almonds with the dried apricots.

3. Spray the bottom and sides of a 2-quart pie dish with canola oil cooking spray. Sprinkle the finely chopped almonds on the base of the dish. Arrange one layer of bread slices on the bottom of the pie dish. The bread slices should fit snugly, so cut accordingly.

4. Sprinkle half of the almond and apricot mixture on top of the bread layer. Repeat step 3 and top again with the remaining almond and apricot mixture.

5. In a large bowl, whisk the eggs, sugar, Splenda, butter and ¼ cup of the mascarpone cheese until very smooth.

6. Add the soy milk and 1½ teaspoons of the almond extract. Pour the liquid over the bread, making sure to saturate all of the bread slices. Transfer the pudding to the refrigerator for 15 minutes.

7. Meanwhile, make the apricot glaze by blending the remaining ¼ cup of the mascarpone cheese, the remaining ½ teaspoon of the almond extract, the

sour cream and the apricot jelly together in a food processor until creamy and smooth.

8. Bake the pudding for 35–40 minutes or until done (the pudding should be moist but not wet in the center). Remove the pudding from the oven and immediately glaze with the sour cream mixture. Allow the glaze to sit for 10 to 15 minutes before serving.

9. To serve, cut pudding into individual squares.

Apple-Spice Crisp

SERVES 8

2 GRAMS SATURATED FAT PER SERVING

Ingredients

Canola oil cooking spray
½ cup old-fashioned oats
1 tablespoon whole-wheat flour
¼ cup toasted wheat germ
¼ cup brown sugar
2 tablespoons butter, cold
¼ cup ground flaxseeds
  (we recommend Barlean's brand)

1 cup raisins
1 cup pecans or walnuts, chopped
1 tablespoon pure vanilla extract
½ teaspoon ground cloves
½ teaspoon cinnamon
2 packets Splenda sugar substitute
5 firm, tart apples (such as Granny Smith)
  cored and sliced into thin rings

Method

1. Preheat the oven to 350 degrees and spray a deep pie dish with canola oil cooking spray.

2. In a medium-size bowl, combine the oats, whole-wheat flour, wheat germ and brown sugar; with two knives or your fingers, work in the butter until crumbly. Mix in the ground flaxseeds.

3. In another bowl, mix the raisins and nuts and then add the vanilla extract, ground cloves, cinnamon and Splenda; mix well.

4. Arrange a single layer of apples on the bottom of the pie dish, then top with a third of the raisin and nut mixture; keep repeating until all of the apples, raisins and nuts are in the pie dish. Finish by spreading the oat mixture evenly on top of the apples.

5. Bake for 35 to 40 minutes or until apples are soft and topping is golden brown.

Chef's Notes

Unlike traditional apple crisp, our version has significantly less butter and is made with one-quarter of the amount of sugar and no refined flour. We love lots of spice in our food, but if you prefer a more mild-flavored apple crisp, you may want to eliminate or reduce the ground cloves. Serve with a small spoonful of all-natural vanilla ice cream or a dollop of fresh whipping cream and a little cinnamon on top.

Chocolate Brownie Apple Nut Cake

Serves 10
2.5 Grams Saturated Fat per Serving

Ingredients

Cake:

Canola oil cooking spray
¼ cup high-oleic canola oil
¼ cup unsweetened applesauce
½ cup brown sugar
½ cup Splenda sugar substitute
2 eggs
¼ cup *whole* milk
1 teaspoon pure vanilla extract

½ cup unsweetened cocoa powder
  (such as Ghirardelli)
1 teaspoon instant espresso
1 cup whole wheat flour
1 teaspoon baking soda
⅛ teaspoon salt
2 apples, peeled and chopped
1 cup walnuts, finely chopped

Frosting:

½ cup whipped cream cheese
½ cup powdered sugar
½ cup Splenda sugar substitute
½ cup unsweetened cocoa powder
  (such as Ghirardelli)

2 teaspoons vanilla extract
2 tablespoons light sour cream

Cake:

1. Preheat the oven to 325 degrees. Spray the bottom of a 9-inch round or square baking pan with canola oil cooking spray.

2. Beat the canola oil, applesauce, brown sugar and Splenda. Beat in the eggs, milk and vanilla extract.

3. In a separate bowl, combine the cocoa powder, espresso, whole-wheat flour, soda and salt. Add the dry ingredients to the wet ingredients and mix thoroughly. Stir in the apples and nuts and pour into the prepared pan.

4. Bake for 40 to 45 minutes. Remove from oven and allow brownie-cake to cool in the pan (you can refrigerate to speed the process along). When brownie-cake is completely cool, spread the frosting on the top (decorate with additional walnuts if desired).

Frosting:

Mix all of the frosting ingredients together in a medium-size bowl and beat with an electric blender until smooth and creamy.

Chocolate-Covered Peanut Buttery Balls

SERVES 18 (1 BALL = 1 SERVING)
2 GRAMS SATURATED FAT PER SERVING

Ingredients

1 cup all-natural (must contain
  no hydrogenated oil) chunky
  peanut butter
½ cup dry nonfat powdered milk
1 cup finely chopped peanuts
  (save time and buy prechopped nuts)

1 tablespoon molasses
½ cup old-fashioned rolled oats
4 ounces semisweet chocolate
  chips (such as Ghirardelli)

Method

1. Mix the peanut butter, powdered milk, peanuts, molasses and oats. Roll mixture into 1-inch balls and place on a large flat platter or cookie sheet.

2. Place the chocolate chips in a microwave-safe dish and heat until just melted, stir and then spoon the melted chocolate on top of the peanut butter balls. **Note:** *Do not coat the entire ball with chocolate, only coat the tops.*

3. Refrigerate for 1½ hours and serve.

Chef's Notes

Busy moms will love these no-bake treats. Our son's best friend's mom gave us this recipe and the kids go nuts for it—Mom and Dad do, too!

Lemony Pecan Bites

SERVES 20

1.5 GRAMS SATURATED FAT PER COOKIE

Ingredients

Canola oil cooking spray
¼ cup butter, softened to
   room temperature
⅓ cup high-oleic canola oil
¼ cup pure maple syrup
½ cup Splenda sugar substitute

2 cups whole-wheat pastry flour
1 teaspoon pure vanilla extract
1 tablespoon fresh lemon juice
1½ cups pecans, finely chopped
   (buy prechopped pecans to save time)

Method

1. Preheat the oven to 325 degrees and spray two baking sheets with canola oil cooking spray.

2. In a large bowl use an electric mixer to cream the butter, oil and maple syrup. Add the Splenda. Mix the flour in a little bit at a time; add in the vanilla extract and lemon juice. Stir in the chopped pecans.

3. Form the dough into 1-inch balls and place on the prepared baking sheets. Press the dough to flatten somewhat and bake for 25 minutes.

4. Let the cookies cool for 10 to 15 minutes before serving.

Chef's Notes

Indulge guilt free! Not only do these cookies taste amazing, they're really not that bad for you; they're rich in fiber, low in sugar, low in saturated fat and high in heart-healthy monounsaturated fat.

Luscious Pumpkin Cheesecake

SERVES 14

3.2 GRAMS SATURATED FAT PER SERVING

Ingredients

Crust:

¾ cup wheat germ

2 tablespoons applesauce

2 teaspoons high-oleic canola oil

1 teaspoon allspice

Filling:

8 ounces Neufchâtel cream cheese

8 ounces fat-free cream cheese

¼ cup firmly packed brown sugar

¼ cup honey

¼ cup Splenda sugar substitute

1 cup canned pumpkin

1 teaspoon pure vanilla extract

2 teaspoons cinnamon

¼ teaspoon ground cloves

½ cup low-fat milk

4 whole eggs

2 egg whites

Method

Crust:

1. Preheat oven to 350 degrees.

2. In a medium-size bowl, mix wheat germ, applesauce, canola oil and all-spice.

3. Place wheat germ mixture in the bottom of a 10-inch springform pan, pressing firmly to cover the bottom of the pan. Bake for 15 minutes. Remove from oven and cool slightly.

Filling:

1. Cream the two cream cheeses, brown sugar, honey and Splenda in a large mixing bowl. Add canned pumpkin, vanilla, cinnamon, ground cloves, milk, eggs and egg whites. Using an electric mixer, blend on medium-high speed until smooth and creamy (mixture should be lump-free).

2. Reset oven to 300 degrees. Pour cream cheese filling into prebaked pie crust and bake for 1 hour and 30 minutes. Turn the oven off and let cheesecake sit in the oven for an additional hour.

3. Remove from oven and chill for *at least* an hour (or until cold and firm) in the refrigerator. Serve cold.

Nutty Dessert Topping

SERVES 20

0 GRAMS SATURATED FAT PER SERVING

Ingredients

2 egg whites

2 teaspoons water

⅓ cup sugar

1 teaspoon salt

2 teaspoons cinnamon

1½ pound shelled pecans

1½ cups whole-wheat Post Shredded
    Wheat cereal (spoon sized)

Canola oil cooking spray

½ cup Splenda all-natural sugar substitute

Method

1. Preheat oven to 300 degrees.

2. Beat the egg whites and water in a medium-sized bowl. Mix in sugar, salt and cinnamon.

3. Spread the pecans and Post Shredded Wheat cereal on a cookie sheet lined with aluminum foil and sprayed with cooking spray; pour the cinnamon and egg white mixture over the pecan mixture. Mix gently with your hands until the pecans and cereal are well coated.

3. Bake the pecan mixture at 300 degrees for 30–40 minutes (toss gently with a spatula several times during the cooking process).

4. Immediately after removing the pecan mixture from the oven, sprinkle and toss with Splenda.

5. Let the pecan mixture cool completely and sit for at least an hour before serving. Store the Nutty Dessert Topping in an air-tight cookie container. **Note:** *This dessert topping can be made well in advance and stored for up to a week.*

Chef's Notes:

This recipe is wonderful served on ice cream, on top of baked fruit, or simply eaten alone. If eating ice cream, be sure to use all-natural ice cream made without hydrogenated oils, and look for one with no more than 5 grams of saturated fat per serving. Also, be sure to stick to the serving size, which is usually ½ cup (or 4 ounces).

Paradise Prune Squares with Lemon Cream Cheese Frosting

SERVES 15

4.25 GRAMS SATURATED FAT PER SERVING

Ingredients

Squares:

2 cups pitted prunes, lightly cooked
(see directions below)

2 cups whole-wheat flour

1 teaspoon salt

1 teaspoon baking soda

1 teaspoon baking powder

1 teaspoon cinnamon

1 teaspoon allspice

1 teaspoon nutmeg

¼ cup sugar

⅓ cup Splenda sugar substitute

3 eggs

1 teaspoon pure vanilla extract

¼ cup high-oleic canola oil

¼ cup butter, softened

1¼ cups low-fat plain yogurt

1 cup walnuts, chopped

Canola oil cooking spray

Frosting:

3 tablespoons butter, softened

6 tablespoons whipped cream cheese

3 tablespoons powdered sugar

5 tablespoons Splenda sugar substitute

1½ teaspoons grated lemon rind

Method

1. Preheat the oven to 350 degrees.

2. Place the prunes in a small saucepan and add just enough water to cover; cover and bring to a boil. Boil for 8 to 10 minutes or until prunes are soft.

3. Sift and mix the dry ingredients (flour, salt, baking soda, baking powder, spices, sugar and Splenda) into a large bowl.

4. Beat the eggs. Add the vanilla extract, oil, softened butter and the yogurt to the eggs and mix well. Add the egg mixture to the flour mixture. Add the chopped walnuts to the batter and mix well.

5. Drain the prunes and chop into small pieces. Mix the prunes with the batter. Use a hand mixer to blend thoroughly.

6. Line a 13-x-9-inch baking pan with waxed paper and spray the paper with cooking spray. Spread the batter evenly in the pan and bake for about

45 to 50 minutes. When done, turn the cake onto a platter and cool completely before frosting.

7. To make the frosting, use a hand mixer and cream at high speed the softened butter and cream cheese. Add the powdered sugar and Splenda, and continue mixing until well blended. Add the grated lemon rind and mix briefly. Spread a thin layer of frosting on the prune cake and cut into approximately 1-inch squares. **Note:** *If serving to company, you may want to decorate each square with a fresh strawberry.*

Rum Runner's Caribbean Carrot Cake

SERVES: 12

2 GRAMS SATURATED FAT PER SERVING

Ingredients

Cake ingredients:

2 eggs

2 tablespoons honey

¼ cup Splenda sugar substitute

¼ cup high-oleic canola oil

1 teaspoon almond extract

2 tablespoons rum

½ cup unsweetened applesauce

⅓ cup plain low-fat yogurt

2 cups whole wheat flour

1 teaspoon ground cinnamon

1 teaspoon baking soda

1 teaspoon baking powder

⅓ cup white raisins

2 cups shredded carrots (buy
    pre-shredded to save time)

1 cup pecans, finely chopped

Canola oil cooking spray

Glaze ingredients:

1 tablespoon butter, softened at room temperature

¼ cup whipped cream cheese

2 tablespoons rum

½ cup sifted powdered sugar

Method

Cake:

1. Preheat oven to 350 degrees.

2. In a large mixing bowl, beat together the eggs, honey, Splenda, canola oil, almond extract, rum, applesauce, and yogurt. Mix in the whole wheat flour, cinnamon, baking soda and baking powder. Stir in the raisins, carrots, and chopped pecans.

3. Generously spray an 8-inch square glass baking pan liberally with canola oil cooking spray and dust lightly with flour. Pour cake mixture into pan and smooth the top evenly with a knife.

4. Bake cake at 350 degrees for 45 minutes. Remove from oven when a toothpick inserted in the middle comes out clean; then immediately loosen sides and turn out on a cake plate. Place cake in freezer to begin cooling process as cake must be completely cooled before frosting.

Glaze:

1. Beat softened butter with whipped cream cheese on highest speed with electric mixer until light and fluffy. Add rum and powdered sugar and continue beating on high speed until fluffy. Use a knife to frost the top of the cake. Decorate cake with small marzipan carrots, candy carrots, or pecan halves.

Conclusion

He who has health has hope,
and he who has hope has everything.
Arabian Proverb

We hope reading the Cure has given you a positive outlook on your future health. Whether you want to lose ten pounds or one hundred pounds, lower your cholesterol, reduce your risk of heart disease and cancer, control your diabetes, increase your energy levels, or improve one of the many inflammatory-mediated conditions we have discussed, following the Gold Coast Cure will undoubtedly improve your health and the health of your loved ones. The Cure is the lifestyle plan your entire family can confidently follow together, in sickness and in health.

We truly hope we have motivated you to ditch dieting and instead make permanent lifestyle changes. We also hope you are convinced that you don't need to deprive yourself of great-tasting food, nor do you need to spend hours at the gym to dramatically improve your health and appearance. The Gold Coast Cure is a realistic lifestyle makeover you can commit to for life—for your life. The rewards will be well worth the initial effort. This we promise.

To contact Andy and Ivy go to:
www.goldcoastcure.com
www.goldcoastsurgery.com

Endnotes

Introduction

1. Weinshenker BG. "Epidemiology of multiple sclerosis." *Neurol Clin.* 1996 May; 14(2): 291–308.
2. Bates D, et al. "A double-blind controlled trial of long chain n–3 polyunsaturated fatty acids in the treatment of multiple sclerosis." *J Neurol Neurosurg Psychiatry.* 1989 Jan; 52(1): 18–22.
3. Nordvik I, et al. "Effect of dietary advice and n–3 supplementation in newly diagnosed MS patients." *Acta Neurol Scand.* 2000 Sep; 102(3): 143–9.
4. Gallai V, et al. "Cytokine secretion and eicosanoid production in the peripheral blood mononuclear cells of MS patients undergoing dietary supplementation with n–3 polyunsaturated fatty acids." *J Neuroimmunol.* 1995 Feb; 56(2): 143–53.
5. Esparza ML, et al. "Nutrition, latitude, and multiple sclerosis mortality: an ecologic study." *Am J Epidemiol.* 1995 Oct 1; 142(7): 733–7.

Chapter 1

1. Foster GD, et al. "A randomized trial of a low-carbohydrate diet for obesity." *N Engl J Med.* 2003 May 22; 348(21); 2082–90.
2. "Letter Report on Dietary Reference Intakes for Trans Fatty Acids." Institute of Medicine, 2002, July 10.
3. de Roos NM, et al. "Replacement of dietary saturated fatty acids by trans fatty acids lowers serum HDL cholesterol and impairs endothelial function in healthy men and women." *Arterioscler Thromb Vasc Biol.* 2001 Jul; 21(7): 1233–7.
4. Willett WC, et al. "Intake of trans fatty acids and risk of coronary heart disease among women." *Lancet.* 1993 Mar 6; 341(8845): 581–5.
5. Ascherio A, et al. "Trans fatty acids and coronary heart disease." Department of Nutrition and Epidemiology, Harvard School of Public Health, 1999.

6. Han SN, et al. "Effect of hydrogenated and saturated, relative to polyunsaturated, fat on immune and inflammatory responses of adults with moderate hypercholesterolemia." *J Lipid Res.* 2002 Mar; 43(3): 445–52.

7. Fried SK, Rao SP. "Sugars, hypertriglyceridemia, and cardiovascular disease." *Am J Clin Nutr.* 2003 Oct; 78(4): 873S–880S.

8. Jeppesen J, et al. "Relation of high TG-low HDL cholesterol and LDL cholesterol to the incidence of ischemic heart disease. An 8-year follow-up in the Copenhagen Male Study." *Arterioscler Thromb Vasc Biol.* 1997 Jun; 17(6): 1114–20.

9. Cullen P. "Evidence that triglycerides are an independent coronary heart disease risk factor." *Am J Cardiol.* 2000 Nov 1; 86(9): 943–9.

10. Hu FB, Willett WC. "Optimal Diets for Prevention of Coronary Heart Disease." *JAMA.* 2002 Nov 27; 288(20): 2569–78.

11. Misciagna G, et al. "Diet, physical activity, and gallstones—a population-based, case-control study in southern Italy." *Am J Clin Nutr.* 1999 Jan; 69(1): 120–6.

12. Swank RL, Dugan BB. "Effect of low saturated fat diet in early and late cases of multiple sclerosis." *Lancet.* 1990 Jul 7; 336(8706): 37–9.

13. Huang SL, Pan WH. "Dietary fats and asthma in teenagers: analyses of the first Nutrition and Health Survey in Taiwan (NAHSIT)." *Clin Exp Allergy.* 2001 Dec; 31(12): 1875–80.

14. Erasmus, U. *Fats That Heal, Fats That Kill.* Burnaby, BC, Canada: Alive Books; 1993.

15. van Marken Lichtenbelt WD, et al. "The effect of fat composition of the diet on energy metabolism." *Z Ernahrungswiss.* 1997 Dec; 36(4): 303–5.

16. Cordain L, et al. "Acne vulgaris: a disease of Western civilization." *Arch Dermatol.* 2002 Dec; 138(12): 1584–90.

17. Fairley J, Stacey S. *Feel Fabulous Forever.* Woodstock, NY: The Overlook Press; 1999.

18. Hay AW, et al. "Essential fatty acid restriction inhibits vitamin D-dependent calcium absorption." *Lipids.* 1980 Apr; 15(4): 251–4.

19. Kruger MC, et al. "Calcium, gamma-linolenic acid, and eicosapentaenoic acid supplementation in senile osteoporosis." *Aging* (Milano). 1998 Oct; 10(5): 385–94.

20. Simopoulos AP. "The importance of the ratio of omega–6/omega–3 essential fatty acids." *Biomed Pharmacother.* 2002 Oct; 56(8): 365–79.

21. Slattery ML, et al. "Plant foods, fiber, and rectal cancer." *Am J Clin Nutr.* 2004 Feb; 79(2): 274–81.

22. Aldoori WH, et al. "A prospective study of dietary fiber types and symptomatic diverticular disease in men." *J Nutr.* 1998 Apr; 128(4): 714–9.

23. Howarth NC, et al. "Dietary fiber and weight regulation." *Nutr Rev.* 2001 May; 59(5): 129–39.

24. Alfieri MA, et al. "Fiber intake of normal weight, moderately obese, and severely obese subjects." *Obes Res.* 1995 Nov; 3(6): 541–7.

25. McCann SE, et al. "Risk of human ovarian cancer is related to dietary intake of selected nutrients, phytochemicals, and food groups." *J Nutr.* 2003 Jun; 133(6): 1937–42.

Chapter 2

1. Rein D, et al. "Cocoa inhibits platelet activation and function." *Am J Clin Nutr.* 2000 Jul; 72(1): 30–5.

2. Lee KW, et al. "Cocoa has more phenolic phytochemicals and a higher antioxidant capacity than teas and red wine." *J Agric Food Chem.* 2003 Dec 3; 51(25): 7292–5.

Chapter 3

1. Willett WC, Ascherio A. "Trans fatty acids: are the effects only marginal." *Am J Pub Health.* 1994 May; 84(5): 722–4.

2. Ascherio A, et al. "Trans-fatty acids intake and risk of myocardial infarction." *Circulation.* 1994 Jan; 89(1): 94–101.

3. Blair SN, et al. "Incremental reduction of serum total cholesterol and low-density lipoprotein cholesterol with the addition of a plant stanol ester-containing spread to statin therapy." *Am J Cardiol.* 2000 Jul 1; 86(1): 46–52.

4. Zemel MB. "Role of dietary calcium and dairy products in modulating adiposity." *Lipids.* 2003 Feb; 38(2): 139–46.

5. McNamara DJ. "The impact of egg limitations on coronary heart disease risk: do the numbers add up." *J Am Coll Nutr.* 2000 Oct; 19(Suppl): 540S–548S.

6. Dawber TR, et al. "Eggs, serum cholesterol, and coronary heart disease." *Am J Clin Nutr.* 1982 Oct; 36(4): 617–25.

7. Moeller SM, et al. "The potential role of dietary xanthophylls in cataract and age-related macular degeneration." *J Am Coll Nutr.* 2000 Oct; 19(5Suppl): 522S–527S.

8. Jiang Z, Sim JS. "Consumption of n–3 polyunsaturated fatty acid-enriched eggs and changes in plasma lipids of human subjects." *Nutrition.* 1993 Nov-Dec; 9(6): 513–8.

Chapter 4

1. Stevinson C, et al. "Garlic for treating hypercholesterolemia. A meta-analysis of randomized controlled trials." *Ann Intern Med.* 2000 Sep 19; 133(6): 420–9.

2. Kohlmeier L, et al. "Lycopene and myocardial infarction risk in the EURAMIC study." *Am J Epidemiol.* 1997 Oct 15; 146(8): 618–26.
3. Fowke JH, et al. "Brassica vegetable consumption shifts estrogen metabolism in healthy postmenopausal women." *Cancer Epidemiol Biomarkers Prev.* 2000 Aug; 9(8): 773–9.
4. Poulter N, et al. "Lipid profiles after the daily consumption of an oat-based cereal: a controlled crossover trial." *Am J Clin Nutr.* 1994 Jan; 59(1): 66–9.

Chapter 5

1. McCann SC, et al. "The risk of breast cancer associated with dietary lignans differs by CYP17 genotype in women." *J Nutr.* 2002 Oct; 132(10): 3036–41.
2. Horn-Ross PL, et al. "Phytoestrogen intake and endometrial cancer risk." *J Natl Cancer Inst.* 2003 Aug 6; 95(15): 1158–64.
3. Strom SS, et al. "Phytoestrogen intake and prostate cancer: a case-control study using a new database." *Nutr Cancer.* 1999; 33(1): 20–5.
4. Almario RU, et al. "Effects of walnut consumption on plasma fatty acids and lipoproteins in combined hyperlipidemia." *Am J Clin Nutr.* 2001 Jul; 74(1): 72–9.
5. Curb JD, et al. "Serum lipid effects of a high-monounsaturated fat diet based on macadamia nuts." *Arch Intern Med.* 2000 Apr 24; 160(8): 1154–8.
6. Rajaram S, et al. "A monounsaturated fatty acid-rich pecan–enriched diet favorably alters the serum lipid profile of healthy men and women." *J Nutr.* 2001 Sep; 131(9): 2275–9.
7. Jiang R, et al. "Nut and peanut butter consumption and risk of type 2 diabetes in women." *JAMA.* 2002 Nov 27; 288(20): 2254–60.
8. Sabate J. "Nut consumption and body weight." *Am J Clin Nutr.* 2003 Sep; 78(3 Suppl): 647S–650S.
9. Hu FB, Stampfer MJ. "Nut consumption and risk of coronary heart disease: a review of epidemiologic evidence." *Curr Atheroscler Rep.* 1999 Nov; 1(3): 204–9.

Chapter 6

1. *Tufts University Health & Nutrition Letter.* Dec 2001.
2. Mozaffarian D, et al. "Cardiac benefits of fish consumption may depend on the type of fish meal consumed: the Cardiovascular Health Study." *Circulation.* 2003 Mar 18; 107(10): 1372–7.
3. von Schackey C, et al. "The effect of dietary omega-3 fatty acids on coronary atherosclerosis. A randomized, double-blind, placebo-controlled trial." *Ann Intern Med.* 1999 Apr 6; 130(7): 554–62.

4. He K, et al. "Fish consumption and risk of stroke in men." *JAMA.* 2002 Dec 25; 288(24): 3130–6.

5. Geleijnse JM, et al. "Blood pressure response to fish oil supplementation: metaregression analysis of randomized trials." *J Hypertens.* 2002 Aug; 20(8): 1493–9.

6. Albert CM, et al. "Blood levels of long chain n–3 fatty acids and the risk of sudden death." *N Engl J Med.* 2002 Apr 11; 346(15): 1113–8.

7. Durrington PN, et al. "An omega-3 polyunsaturated fatty acid concentrate administered for one year decreased triglycerides in simvastatin treated patients with coronary heart disease and persisting hypertriglyceridemia." *Heart.* 2001 May; 85(5): 544–8.

8. Okuda Y, et al. "Long-term effects of eicosapentaenoic acid on diabetic peripheral neuropathy and serum lipids in patients with type II diabetes mellitus." *J Diabetes Complications.* 1996 Sep-Oct; 10(5): 280–7.

9. Hu FB, et al. "Fish and long-chain omega-3 fatty acid intake and risk of coronary heart disease and total mortality in diabetic women." *Circulation.* 2003 Apr 15; 107(14): 1852–7.

10. Sirtori CR, et al. "N–3 fatty acids do not lead to an increased diabetic risk in patients with hyperlipidemia and abnormal glucose tolerance. Italian Fish Oil Multicenter Study." *Am J Clin Nutr.* 1997 Jun; 65(6): 1874–81.

11. Dunstan DW, et al. "The independent and combined effects of aerobic exercise and dietary fish intake on serum lipids and glycemic control in NIDDM. A randomized controlled study." *Diabetes Care.* 1997 Jun; 20(6): 913–21.

12. Bosetti C, et al. "A pooled anaylsis of case-controlled studies of thyroid cancer. VI. Fish and shellfish consumption." *Cancer Causes Control.* 2001 May; 12(4): 375–82.

13. Caygill CP, Hill MJ. "Fish, n–3 fatty acids and human colorectal and breast cancer mortality." *Eur J Cancer Prev.* 1995 Aug; 4(4): 329–32.

14. Norrish AE, et al. "Prostate cancer risk and consumption of fish oils: a dietary biomarker-based case-control study." *Br J Cancer.* 1999 Dec; 81(7): 1238–42.

15. Morris MC, et al. "Consumption of fish and n–3 fatty acids and risk of incident Alzheimer disease." *Arch Neurol.* 2003 Jul; 60(7): 940–6.

16. Mickleborough TD, et al. "Fish oil supplementation reduces severity of exercise-induced bronchoconstriction in elite athletes." *Am J Respir Crit Care Med.* 2003 Nov 15; 168(10): 1181–9.

17. Swank RL, et al. "Multiple sclerosis in rural Norway: its geographic and occupational incidence in relation to nutrition." *N Engl J Med.* 1952 May 8; 246(19): 722–8.

18. Esparza ML, et al. Nutrition, latitude, and multiple sclerosis mortality: an ecologic study." *Am J Epidemiol.* 1995 Oct 1; 142(7): 733–7.

19. Geusens P, et al. "Long-term effect of omega-3 fatty acid supplementation in active rheumatoid arthritis. A 12-month, double-blind, controlled study." *Arthritis Rheum.* 1994 Jun; 37(6): 824–9.

20. Aslan A, Triadafilopoulos G. "Fish oil fatty acid supplementation in active ulcerative colitis: a double-blind, placebo-controlled, crossover study." *Am J Gastroenterol,* 1992 Apr; 87(4): 432–7.

21. Helland IB, et al. "Maternal supplementation with very long chain fatty acids during pregnancy and lactation augments children's IQ at 4 years of age." *Pediatrics.* 2003 Jan; 111(1): e39–44.

22. Stevens LJ, et al. "Omega-3 fatty acids in boys with behavior, learning, and health problems." *Physiol Behav.* 1996 Apr-May; 59(4–5): 915–20.

23. Nagakura T, et al. "Dietary supplementation with fish oil rich in omega-3 polyunsaturated fatty acids in children with bronchial asthma." *Eur Respir J.* 2000 Nov; 16(5): 861–5.

24. Dunstan JA, et al. "Fish oil supplementation in pregnancy modifies neonatal allergen-specific immune responses and clinical outcomes in infants at high risk of atopy: a randomized, controlled trial." *J Allergy Clin Immunol.* 2003 Dec; 112(6): 1178–84.

25. Yoshizawa K, et al. "Mercury and the risk of coronary heart disease in men." *N Engl J Med.* 2002 Nov 28; 347(22): 1755–60.

26. Zhang J, et al. "Fish consumption and mortality from all causes, ischemic heart disease and stroke: an ecological study." *Prev Med.* 1999 May; 28(5): 520–9.

27. Davidson PW, et al. "Effects of prenatal and postnatal methylmercury exposure from fish consumption on neurodevelopment: outcomes at 66 months of age in the Seychelles Child Development Study." *JAMA.* 1998 Aug 26; 280(8): 701–7.

28. Myers GJ, et al. "Prenatal methylmercury exposure from ocean fish consumption in the Seychelles Child Development Study." *Lancet.* 2003 May 17; 361 (9370): 1686–92.

29. Foran SE, et al. "Measurement of mercury levels in concentrated over-the-counter fish oil preparations: is fish oil healthier than fish?" *Arch Pathol Lab Med.* 2003 Dec; 127(12): 1603–5.

30. FAO/WHO/UNU Expert Consultation. Energy and Protein Requirements. 1985, Geneva: World Health Organization. (WHO technical report, series 724).

31. Erdman JW Jr. "AHA Science Advisory: Soy protein and cardiovascular disease: A statement for healthcare professionals from the Nutrition Committee of the AHA." *Circulation.* 2000 Nov 14; 102(20): 2555–9.

32. Anderson JW, et al. "Meta-analysis of the effects of soy protein intake on serum lipids." *N Engl J Med.* 1995 Aug 3; 333(5): 276–82.

33. Liu RH. "Health benefits of fruit and vegetables are from additive and synergistic combinations of phytochemicals." *Am J Clin Nutr.* 2003 Sep; 78(3 Suppl): 517S–520S.

34. Nagata C, et al. "Soy product intake and hot flashes in Japanese women: results from a community-based prospective study." *Am J Epidemiol.* 2001 Apr 15; 153(8): 790–3.

35. Alekel DL, et al. "Isoflavone-rich soy protein isolate attenuates bone loss in the lumbar spine of perimenopausal women." *Am J Clin Nutr.* 2000 Sep; 72(3): 844–52.

36. Morimoto LM. "Obesity, body size, and risk of postmenopausal breast cancer: the Women's Health Initiative (United States)." *Cancer Causes Control.* 2002 Oct; 13(8): 741–51.

37. Dai Q, et al. "Population-based case-control study of soyfood intake and breast cancer risk in Shanghai." *Br J Cancer.* 2001 Aug 3; 85(3): 372–8.

38. Linseisen J, et al. "Dietary phytoestrogen intake and premenopausal breast cancer risk in a German case-control study." *Int J Cancer.* 2004 Jun 10; 110(2): 284–90.

39. Lee MM, et al. "Soy and isoflavone consumption in relation to prostate cancer risk in China." *Cancer Epidemiol Biomarkers Prev.* 2003 Jul; 12(7): 665–8.

40. Hebert JR, et al. "Nutritional and socioeconomic factors in relation to prostate cancer mortality: a cross-national study." *J Natl Cancer Inst.* 1998 Nov 4; 90(21): 1637–47.

Chapter 7

1. Gronbaek M, et al. "Mortality associated with moderate intakes of wine, beer, or spirits." *BMJ.* 1995 May 6; 310(6988): 1165–9.

2. Friedman LA, Kimball AW. "Coronary heart disease mortality and alcohol consumption in Framingham." *Am J Epidemiol.* 1986 Sep; 124(3): 481–9.

3. Truelsen, et al. "Intake of beer, wine, and spirits and risk of stroke: The Copenhagen City Heart Study." *Stroke.* 1998 Dec; 29(12): 2467–72.

4. Sacco RL, et al. "The protective effect of moderate alcohol consumption on ischemic stroke." *JAMA.* 1999 Jan 6; 281(1): 53–60.

5. Mukamal KJ, et al. "Prospective study of alcohol consumption and risk of dementia in older adults." *JAMA.* 2003 Mar 19; 289(11): 1405–13.

6. Zuccala G, et al. "Dose-related impact of alcohol consumption on cognitive function in advanced age: results of a multicenter survey." *Alcohol Clin Exp Res.* 2001 Dec; 25(12): 1743–8.

7. Orgogozo JM, et al. "Wine consumption and dementia in the elderly; a prospective community study in the Bordeaux area." *Rev Neurol (Paris)*. 1997 Apr; 153(3): 185–92.

8. Davies MJ, et al. "Effects of moderate alcohol intake on fasting insulin and glucose concentrations and insulin sensitivity in postmenopausal women: a randomized controlled trial." *JAMA*. 2002 May 15; 287(19): 2559–62.

9. Stampfer MJ, et al. "A prospective study of moderate alcohol drinking and risk of diabetes in women." *Am J Epidemiol*. 1988 Sep; 128(3): 549–58.

10. Solomon CG, et al. "Moderate alcohol consumption and risk of coronary heart disease among women with type 2 diabetes mellitus." *Circulation*. 2000 Aug 1; 102(5): 494–9.

11. Cordain L, et al. "Influence of moderate daily wine consumption upon body weight regulation and metabolism in healthy free-living males." *J Am Coll Nutr*. 1997 Apr; 16(2): 134–9.

12. Greenfield JR, et al. "Moderate alcohol consumption, dietary fat composition, and abdominal obesity in women: evidence for gene-environment interaction." *J Clin Endocrinol Metab*. 2003 Nov; 88(11): 5381–6.

13. Liu S, et al. "A prospective study of alcohol intake and change in body weight among US adults." *Am J Epidemiol*. 1994 Nov 15; 140(10): 912–20.

14. Kahn HS, et al. "Stable behaviors associated with adults' 10-year change in body mass index and likelihood of gain at the waist." *Am J Public Health*. 1997 May; 87(5): 747–54.

15. Gronbaek M, et al. "Mortality associated with moderate intakes of wine, beer, or spirits." *BMJ*. 1995 May 6; 310(6988): 1165–9.

16. Mukamal KJ, et al. "Roles of drinking pattern and type of alcohol consumed in coronary heart disease in men." *N Engl J Med*. 2003 Jan 9; 348(2): 109–18.

17. Klatsky AL, et al. "Wine, liquor, beer, and mortality." *Am J Epidemiol*. 2003 Sep 15; 158(6): 585–95.

18. Iwai N, et al. "Relationship between coffee and green tea consumption and all-cause mortality in a cohort of a rural Japanese population." *J Epidemiol*. 2002 May; 12(3): 191–8.

19. Salazar-Martinez E, et al. "Coffee consumption and risk for type 2 diabetes mellitus." *Ann Intern Med*. 2004 Jan 6; 140(1): 1–8.

20. Tuomilehto J, et al. "Coffee consumption and risk of type II diabetes mellitus among middle-aged Finnish men and women." *JAMA*. 2004 Mar 10; 291(10): 1213–9.

21. Ross GW, et al. "Association of coffee and caffeine intake with the risk of Parkinson disease." *JAMA*. 2000 May 24–31; 283(20): 2674–9.

22. Willett WC, et al. "Coffee consumption and coronary heart disease in women. A ten year follow-up." *JAMA*. 1996 Feb 14; 275(6): 458–62.

23. Grobbee DE, et al. "Coffee, caffeine and cardiovascular disease in men." *N Engl J Med.* 1990 Oct 11; 323(15): 1026–32.
24. Schwartz J, Weiss ST. "Caffeine intake and asthma symptoms." *Ann Epidemiol.* 1992 Sep; 2(5): 627–35.
25. Pagano R, et al. "Coffee drinking and prevalence of bronchial asthma." *Chest.* 1988 Aug; 94(2): 386–9.
26. Curhan GC, et al. "Beverage use and risk for kidney stones in women." *Ann Intern Med.* 1998 Apr 1; 128(7): 534–40.
27. Leitzmann MF, et al. "Prospective study of coffee consumption and the risk of symptomatic gallstone disease in men" *JAMA.* 1999 Jun 9; 281(22): 2106–12.
28. Yoshida H, et al. "Inhibitory effect of tea flavonoids on the ability of cells to oxidize low density lipoprotein." *Biochem Pharmacol.* 1999 Dec; 58(11): 1695–703.
29. Sesso HD, et al., "Coffee and tea intake and the risk of myocardial infarction." *Am J Epidemiol.* 1999 Jan 15; 149(2): 162–7.
30. Geleijnse JM, et al. "Inverse association of tea and flavonoid intakes with incident myocardial infarction: the Rotterdam study." *Am J Clin Nutr.* 2002 May; 75(5): 880–6.
31. Dora I, et al. "Black tea consumption and risk of rectal cancer in Moscow population." *Ann Epidemiol.* 2003 Jul; 13(6): 405–11.
32. Wu AH, et al. "Green tea and risk of breast cancer in Asian Americans." *Int J Cancer.* 2003 Sep 10; 106(4): 574–9.
33. Dulloo AG, et al. "Efficacy of a green tea extract rich in catechin polyphenols and caffeine in increasing 24–h energy expenditure and fat oxidation in humans." *Am J Clin Nutr.* 1999 Dec; 70(6): 1040–5.

Chapter 10

1. Blumenthal JA, et al. "Exercise and weight loss reduce blood pressure in men and women with mild hypertension: effects on cardiovascular, metabolic, and hemodynamic functioning." *Arch Intern Med.* 2000 Jul 10; 160(13): 1947–58.
2. Wood PD, et al. "The effects on plasma lipoproteins of a prudent weight-reducing diet, with or without exercise, in overweight men and women." *N Engl J Med.* 1991 Aug 15; 325(7): 461–6.
3. Province MA, et al. "The effects of exercise on falls in elderly patients. A pre-planned meta-analysis of the FICSIT trials. Frailty and Injuries: Cooperative Studies of Intervention Techniques." *JAMA.* 1995 May 3; 273(17): 1341–7.
4. Baker KR, et al. "The efficacy of home based progressive strength training in older adults with knee osteoarthritis: a randomized controlled trial." *J Rheumatol.* 2001 Jul; 28(7): 1655–65.

5. Richards SC, Scott DL. "Prescribed exercise in people with fibromyalgia: parallel group randomized controlled trial." *BMJ*. 2002 Jul 27; 325(7357): 185.

6. Wallman KE, et al. "Randomised controlled trial of graded exercise in chronic fatigue syndrome." *Med J Aust*. 2004 May 3; 180(9): 444–8.

7. McTiernan A, et al. "Recreational physical activity and the risk of breast cancer in postmenoupausal women: the Women's Health Initiative Cohort Study." *JAMA*. 2003 Sep 10; 290(10): 1331–6.

8. Castaneda C, et al. "A randomized controlled trial of resistance exercise training to improve glycemic control in older adults with type 2 diabetes." *Diabetes Care*. 2002 Dec; 25(12): 2335–41.

9. Bryner RW, et al. "Effects of resistance vs. aerobic training combined with an 800 calorie liquid diet on lean body mass and resting metabolic rate." *J Am Coll Nutr*. 1999 Apr; 18(2): 115–21.

Chapter 11

1. Fletcher RH, Fairfield KM. "Vitamins for chronic disease prevention in adults: clinical applications." *JAMA*. 2002 Jun 19; 287(23): 3127–9.

2. Ruml LA, et al. "The effect of calcium citrate on bone density in the early and mid-postmenopausal period: a randomized placebo-controlled study." *Am J Ther*. 1999 Nov; 6(6): 303–11.

3. Kampman E, et al. "Calcium, vitamin D, sunshine exposure, dairy products and colon cancer risk (United States)." *Cancer Causes Control*. 2000 May; 11(5): 459–66.

4. Zemel MB. "Regulation of adiposity and obesity risk by dietary calcium: mechanisms and implications." *J Am Coll Nutr*. 2002 Apr; 21(2): 146S–151S.

5. Shapses SA, et al. "Effect of calcium supplementation on weight and fat loss in women." *J Clin Endocrinol Metab*. 2004 Feb; 89(2): 632–7.

6. Munger KL, et al. "Vitamin D intake and multiple sclerosis" *Neurology*. 2004 Jan 13; 62(1): 60–5.

7. Kawano Y, et al. "Effects of magnesium supplementation in hypertensive patients: assessment by office, home, and ambulatory blood pressures." *Hypertension*. 1998 Aug; 32(2): 260–5.

8. Zandi PP, et al. "Reduced risk of Alzheimer's disease in users of antioxidant vitamin supplements: the Cache County study." *Arch Neurol*. 2004 Jan; 61(1): 82–8.

9. Miller ER, et al. "Meta-Analysis: High-Dosage Vitamin E Supplementation May Increase All Cause-Mortality." *Ann Intern Med*. 2004 Nov 10; Epub ahead of print.

10. Knekt P, et al. "Serum selenium and subsequent risk of cancer among Finnish men and women." *J Natl Cancer Inst*. 1990 May 16; 82(10): 864–8.

11. Salonen RM, et al. "Six-year effect of combined vitamin C and E supplementation on atherosclerotic progression: the Antioxidant Supplementation in Atherosclerosis Prevention (ASAP) Study." *Circulation.* 2003 Feb 25; 107(7): 947–53.
12. Keen H, et al. "Treatment of diabetic neuropathy with gamma-linolenic acid. The gamma-Linolenic Acid Multicenter Trial Group." *Diabetes Care.* 1993 Jan; 16(1): 8–15.
13. Ishikawa T., et al. "Effects of gammalinolenic acid on plasma lipoproteins and apolipoproteins" *Atherosclerosis.* 1989 Feb; 75(2–3): 95–104.

Index